Intuitive Eating

by Lucia Bartoli

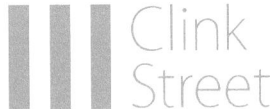
Clink Street

Published by Clink Street Publishing 2022

ISBN:
978-1-915229-55-7 - paperback
978-1-915229-56-4 - ebook

Contents

The Forbidden Fruit

Once upon a time, in the beginning of time, there lived a young boy and a young girl. They lived in a beautiful land, a magical forest-like place. Where it was always perfectly warm so they needn't wear clothes, the grass was always green and soft to walk on, so they never wore shoes, and the sky was always blue with plenty of sunshine, which helped the plants and trees to flourish all year round with glorious fruits and vegetables, so they never had to worry about food. They called it, The Garden of Eden, and their names, were Adam and Eve. They lived there together just the two of them, they had no stress, no worries, and no fears. There was just one condition, a very simple condition, an easy rule to follow and it was the only rule there was in this mystical land. 'Do not eat the apples from this tree,' they had been told, referring to an apple tree close by. This was the only tree in the whole of the forest which was off-limits. It had a signpost and everything. But somehow, this one rule wasn't sitting quite right with Eve, although the apples from this tree looked no different from all the other apple trees out there, there was just something that bit more appealing about this one. She couldn't quite put her finger on what exactly it was, but in her head, all she kept repeating to herself was 'I mustn't eat those apples, I mustn't eat those apples.' She stopped sleeping at night because all she could think about were those damn apples. Until one night, she got up from her bed of palm leaves and flower petals, and went and sat on a log near by the forbidden tree. Starring up at it, she couldn't help but wonder what it was that was so tempting about it. She already had everything she could ever dream of and other than the fact that she had to populate the world with her brother, her life was pretty much perfect. But at last, the temptation of the forbidden fruit got the better of her. She picked the biggest, reddest, shiniest apple she could see, and took the biggest bite she could possibly take from it, and from that moment on, so the story goes, the perfect world as she knew it, was never to be the same again.

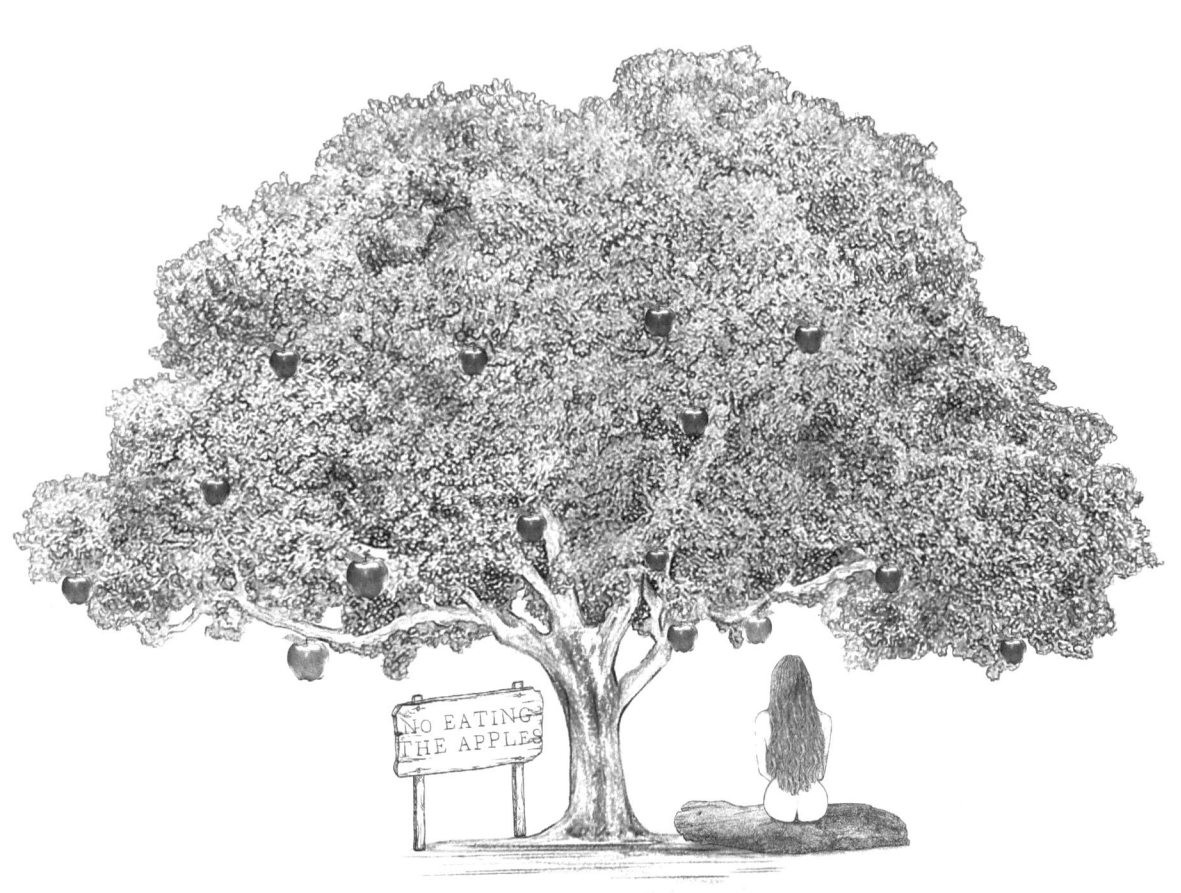

Introduction

This book was written in the hope of inspiring others to take on a new, more valuable, mentality when it comes to eating and self-love. As a 28-year-old woman growing up in the 21st century, I think I can vouch for pretty much *all* women when I say it's not easy. I mean technically, life is easier than ever. It's easier to travel, keep in touch with people, women have more rights now than ever before, but somehow, there's still a certain type of pressure. A pressure that I presume has pretty much always been there (or at least for very long time), and for some reason the weight of this pressure seems to fall much heavier on the shoulders of women. It's the pressure for us to look a certain way, to maintain a certain weight in order to 'fit in', to have the ability to 'snap back' into shape after baring and birthing a child and to present ourselves in a way which is visually pleasing to others. Now in 2022, the world can sometimes give the impression that it's more accepting of different body types, with more plus size models than ever before (which don't get me wrong it great), what was once a size 0 dominated world has now embraced being thick to be the new cool (but even then, it's only *really* acceptable if you're thick in what's deemed as the 'right' places). My point is, there's always been an immense number of expectations and judgments on the female body and it doesn't feel like it's going to change anytime soon. And again, I'd like to take to the liberty of speaking on behalf of the female population when I say, I'm sick of it. Although I had always had somewhat of a love/hate relationship with my body in the past and was always willing to do what it took to fit in with the expectations that were so unwillingly thrust upon me as a young girl growing up, my interest in health, food and nutrition also grew. So I began to read books on the subjects, learnt to cook and educated myself. These books on health and nutrition of course being written mostly by professionals like doctors and scientists. I just couldn't help but feel so disconnected from the authors. They were just so, unrelatable? How could these middle aged (mostly male) doctors and scientists possibly understand how it feels to be a young woman living in these modern times. We can have all the knowledge in the world on food, nutrition and the body, but perhaps what is more important is how we use that knowledge. We can use it to support what seems like an endless cycle of fad diets, weight loss products and withhold the tradition of the diet culture. Or, we can promote a new way of living which is focussed primarily on our health. A mentality which we can pass down to our children and so forth, ultimately making a lasting difference not only to the way which we are physically perceived, but also to how we feel. And that's what drove me to write this book, to share with you all what exactly helped me break free from these pressures of society, a change in psychology which enabled me to live my life in a way which benefited both my physical and mental health. It's something that I wish I would have read a book about when I was younger, it would have saved me a lot of stress, unhealthy diets and unnecessary cosmetic procedures.

In this book you will learn how to rewire old eating habits, change old ways of thinking and to break free from old diet methods which no longer, and have never, served you.

Breaking Free

As we go through life we pick up different traits, beliefs and habits. We're taught these things from the outside world, influenced mostly by a combination of our upbringing and our environment. For example, eating our local cuisine, eating meat because we were brought up eating meat, insecurities about our appearance due to any comments that have been made by others. These are all taught behaviours and all these experiences shape us, we become them. We then further shape our mindsets with the tv shows we watch, the music we listen to, the images we feed ourselves on social media, and the people we choose to hang out with. We're detached from our beings and our true selves because we were never taught how to connect with them in the first place. We were taught from tradition, by people who have their own beliefs and habits, who were raised by others with *their* own beliefs and habits, and the chain goes on. So we too do things out of habit – i.e., mindless eating or eating things because we think we're *supposed* to – 'I have to eat salad because I need to lose some weight' and 'I cannot eat butter as it will make me fat.' We punish ourselves when we do something that goes against these beliefs by speaking badly to ourselves – 'I'm so fat, I'll never lose weight,' and then we force

ourselves to make choices in the future that we know we don't really want to commit to – 'From this day forward no more sugar.' We even judge other people for being different to us – 'She's so skinny she must have an eating disorder' or 'How can she let herself eat like that it's embarrassing.'

These days, you could say pretty much everyone's 'environment' is social media, it's a communal place for people from all over the world. Photos are shared, judgments are made, and the pressure increases. The pressure to become the 'perfect image' we all strive for. In effect, the standards that we've been raised with have now been amplified x1000. It's no longer just you, your family, your community, now the whole world is watching. At this point we've *totally* lost touch with ourselves (if we ever were in touch with them in the first place that is!). You do your best to look absolutely flawless to everyone else, but all that will never make a difference because as long as you hold onto these same old beliefs and habits, you will always be chasing the unrealistic image of perfection.

Most of us want to lose weight to be skinny, and that's it. Just to be skinny. Oh, and also to look good in pictures. And to post them. But that's about as far as it goes. We don't really care how we get there, just as long as the end result is skinny. But by practicing Intuitive Eating, we shift our intention. We let go of our old ways and we are willing to change. We replace *skinny* with *healthy*, we replace seeking approval with self-acceptance, and we replace tradition with open mindedness. Our old mindless *and yet overthinking* ways become filled with awareness, as we begin enjoying life more in the present.

Why should our health prioritise our weight? The answer is this – A person's weight does not determine their health but their health *does* determine their weight. '*Skinny*' does not necessarily mean '*healthy*'. However, someone who is in 'good health' will automatically be in 'good shape'. One of the fastest and most impactful ways to good health is through our diet. In fact, it's said that most illness can be rooted down to diet. As Dr. Michael Greger states in his bestselling book, *How Not To Die*. 'The primary reason diseases tend to run in families may be that diets tend to run in families.'

Roughly every nine years, every cell in our body has been replaced. How crazy to think that you are physically a completely different person than you were nine years ago. The only thing that remains the same is your genetic code (your DNA). When we're born, our bodies are made up solely of our parents and our microbiome, and from that day forward, any new cells we produce or accumulate are made up primarily from two things, 1. (and predominantly) what we put into our bodies (e.g. food and drink), and 2. our environment. So, we literally *are* what we eat. Which also means that any illnesses/diseases that we contract (that aren't completely genetic), are also likely to be created or provoked from this. Even some genetic diseases can be helped or avoided completely just by 'Let(ting) food be thy medicine and medicine be thy food' – Hippocrates (400 BC) Finding a healthy, sustainable way of eating is one of, if not the most important thing when it comes to living a long, healthy and fulfilling life.

But before we make any changes to ourselves we must first become conscious of who we currently are, and only then can we decide who we want to be. We may think we know ourselves but the truth is, most of us are walking around in a total bubble. A bubble of self-conscious, self-critical, judgmental, and *unconscious* behaviour. This bubble acts as a type of shield from the outer world, we even believe it's keeping us safe. And when we look through our bubble onto the outside world it's like looking through a lens, but the lens is like one of those funny mirrors you get at the fun fair, what you're seeing is a distorted reality. It's a reality which has been warped by your beliefs and opinions. Of course, this was bound to happen, we've been raised with this set of values from birth, how could we be any other way?

If you're currently reading this and thinking maybe it doesn't apply to you, ask yourself the following questions:

Do I spend time worrying about what I eat?

Do I ever feel guilty about what I've eaten?

Do I fear/greatly rely on the opinion of others?

Do I lack self-control?

Am I fully aware of my thoughts and behaviour?

If you've answered yes to any of the first four questions, then you too are in a bubble. If you answered yes to fearing the opinion of others then through the lens everyone is a judge to you. If you answered yes to worrying about what you eat, then through the lens every meal time is filled with anxious significance and potential regret. If you answered yes to lacking self-control then through the lens the outside world seems stronger than you are and you are controlled by situations instead of being in control.

The last question however, is a little bit different. If you've answered yes, please be sure that your answer is really a yes. To test this, ask yourself what was the last thing you were thinking of. Do you remember? Whenever you receive a new thought are you aware of it, or do you get caught up in it until the next thought comes along? Are you always aware of how you feel? Are you aware of your posture? Are you aware of your senses, the current smell around you, the sounds, what you can see? Are you aware of the present moment? Are you aware of your eating habits? You might say, 'I'm totally aware of everything I eat, I always read all the ingredients, count every calorie, know exactly the amount of fat and sugar and everything is completely controlled' BUT are you aware that you're now *overthinking*?

There're a million things to be aware of, and we can't be aware of all of them at once. For example, my awareness is currently directed at writing this book so I'm less aware of the smell of my house and the sounds around me. To be completely aware of everything at all times is some *serious* buddha shit. But you don't have to be a buddha to reach inner happiness and contentment with food. You just have to be aware enough to burst your bubble.

This bubble however, doesn't burst so easily, it's taken a long time to grow this protective yet misconstrued filter of *unreasonable* opinions. And you're most likely comfortable in it. You're hard on yourself because it keeps you from acting in a way that's not deemed as acceptable in the future. You avoid certain foods and social events completely because it's easier than facing the fear of lacking control. You encourage yourself with a reward when you conform, you punish yourself when you don't, and you even judge others for not sharing these beliefs. We can't simply burst a whole complex organisation of co-dependent thoughts and beliefs overnight. So instead of bursting the bubble, we become *aware* of the bubble. And then eventually, it will begin to melt away. You know, like those desserts in the fancy restaurants, with the big round chocolate bubble, and the waiter comes and pours the hot chocolate sauce onto it, and it melts away to reveal a glorious, delicious, chocolate cake inside. You are the delicious chocolate cake, you just need to melt your bubble.

As you listen to your body more and learn to become one with it again, you'll feel your intentions will naturally divert.

Make a mental note of where you're at before reading this book, how you feel about yourself, your relationship with food and your general mindset. Better yet, write it down. Then, in a couple of months, after following the advice given to you in here, compare how you feel. Like most things, the longer you practice Intuitive Eating the more you will feel the benefits. This is because, as it becomes a way of life for you, you will change and grow in an amazing way, and the longer it goes on for, the more fulfilling it gets. There really is no end to it. You just keep progressing, feeling better and better. Growing in health, happiness and contentment. Be sure to give yourself time to adjust, it may feel alien to you at first and you'll need to get used to such a big change in mindset. It's normal to feel a bit bumpy and confused in the beginning, but kind of like sailing a boat, once you get past the waves at the shore and sail further into the depths of the ocean, you'll find it begins to feel much smoother. Sure you'll still come across some waves from time to time, but they'll be calmer and far fewer in between, and with more

experience, you'll know exactly how to handle them. From there, positive changes with your body and over-all attitude will follow.

I still have days where I feel myself drifting into old habits and old ways of thinking, and I'm also still learning. But once we realise that just like the waves in ocean will always be there, so will be the temptation of old habits. With this realisation, we then understand that actually, our whole lives are for learning. We 'practice' Intuitive Eating, we 'practice' mediation. It's called a practice because it's always ongoing.

TAKEAWAY

We view the world around us and even our own bodies in a way which we have been taught, and not necessarily how it is.

By following all of what is written in this book I have been able to completely transform my mindset and behavior patterns into ones which allow me to be free to enjoy food, make me healthy and fill me every day with ongoing happiness and a love for life.

This book is about Intuitive Eating. It's not a diet, it's not a fad or a program. It's just you, getting back in touch with you. It's more expansive than any diet, cleanse, treatment or procedure as it effects not only your physical body but your mentality too, in a positive, fulfilling and life-changing way.

Exercise
Noticing your bubble

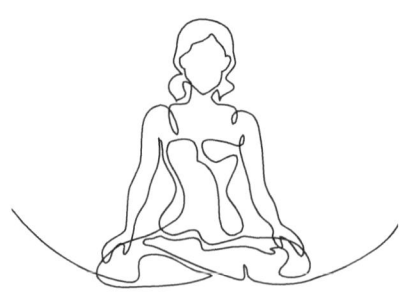

From this moment onwards, I want you to practise this exercise as much as possible. Although it is an 'exercise' the beautiful thing about it is that when practised regularly, it will eventually become completely natural to you.

1. As you go about your day, try to notice your thoughts whenever possible. When you find yourself noticing a thought, simply take the position of a 'viewer' and observe it and let it pass without any forming opinions or attachment to it.

2. Maintain this position of watching your thoughts as much and whenever you can.

——————————————— TIP ———————————————

A good way to help you learn to do this, (a technique I learned from a well-known book called The Untethered Soul by Michael A Singer), is, for one full day, pretend you have a friend in there with you, any thoughts that you hear or see are coming from this friend, and you are just watching and listening to them.

This exercise creates distance between us and our thoughts and by watching them without involving ourselves in them, we are able realise just exactly what our bubbles are made of.

Why we feel the way we do about food

It's hard not to blame ourselves when do things like overeat, I mean, who else's fault could it be? We're the ones with the knife and fork in our hands, we're the ones chewing and swallowing, of course we're the ones to blame? But did you ever stop and ask yourself *why* you feel the way you do when you're eating? Where exactly your strong urge for food comes from? I wanted to take a moment to address these questions because, as you'll read later on in the book, to be an Intuitive Eater, we must learn to forgive ourselves. And to truly be able to forgive ourselves, we must first stop blaming ourselves. To do this, we need to understand just exactly *why* we are the way we are.

Around 70,000 years ago there was an event that scientists named 'the cognitive revolution'. It's a great mystery because, no scientist has ever been able explain just why, or how exactly, this happened. They describe this miraculous change in our brains as a 'genetic glitch'. And this glitch, seems to be the thing that sets us aside from other animals. We developed an awareness that we're yet to see the same levels of in any other species and it's this glitch which allows us to make decisions *consciously*. It allowed us to climb to the top of the food chain (it would usually take millions of years for a species to evolve and make it to the top of the food chain) and pretty much dominate the entire world. It's only since this revolution that our species have been able to successfully spread ourselves around the globe, create art, speak in languages, first speak of religions, build architecture, invent agriculture and farming, and manifest this amazing world that we live in today.

Now if you're asking yourself, what does all this have to with my eating habits? Well, the problem is, even though our brains evolved at a super speed, all of our food-based instincts that took our ancestors millions of years to develop have pretty much remained the same. These instincts developed in very different world to the one we find ourselves in today. In fact, for most of the 300,000 years that our human ancestors have been around, human biologists say that searching for and eating food was a full-time priority (whereas now it's normal to spend more of our energy trying to avoid it!). The most appealing foods being ones higher in calories such as fats (the highest at 9 calories per gram), carbohydrates and protein (both at 4 calories per gram). The reason for this being simple, the more excess calories you eat, the more extra fat your body stores. For our ancestors more fat meant a higher chance of survival through times of famine and scares food. It's no wonder prefer French fries over celery!

When our body's need food, a hormone called ghrelin is released. It's produced predominantly in the stomach and it communicates with the brain to stimulate our appetite giving us that 'hunger' feeling. It's often released around our general meal times and it's released in even greater amounts when we actually see food. Ever been looking at 'food porn' pictures on your phone or an advert on tv and you suddenly feel a bout of hunger which wasn't there before? That's the ghrelin talking. This helped our ancestors survive by letting them know when they're hungry and encouraging them to eat as much as they could when they see food, and in effect, it increased the amount of food they ate and promoted further fat storage. Fast forward a few millennia to the current world we're living in however, and food is *too* accessible. You can literally have any type of food, in any place, at any time. Indian food in London, Mexican food in Italy, tropical fruits in ski resorts and usually, at just the click (or tap) of a finger. It's all too easy, the last thing we then need is further encouragement from big food chains and social media, boosting our Ghrelin levels when we weren't even thinking about food! And so we often find we're in battle with ourselves - our old school instincts vs our newly evolved conscious minds.

So, before you go forward, give yourself a break. It's not actually your fault that you feel the way you do about food. We've evolved to see food and want to eat it, it's literally in our DNA! And it's not just you who has this problem, it's the whole of the human race.

Literally everyone has a built-in desire for food. So why is everyone not obese? Well a largely growing percentage of the population is, but what it boils down to is that some people just feed into these urges more than others (*literally*). While it may seem like we're doomed and there's no way out, rest assured, there is. Because the amazing thing about being a human being is that we are not instinct-driven creatures. We have the ability to contemplate our instincts! Other examples of this are, feeling attracted to the opposite sex, our instincts tell us when we find other people are attractive, and, our thinking brain stops us from sleeping with everyone we find attractive (*it's supposed to anyway*). Our instincts tell us when were tired and want to sleep, but our thinking brain keeps us awake because it knows we're not supposed to be sleeping at 2 pm in the office. Or probably not at all for that matter.

It's important to realise this, it may even sound obvious, but actually the majority of us out there find it hard to differentiate between our instincts and our conscious decisions. When you give your dog a treat you don't see him sitting there staring at it, wondering if it's gluten free, or go to look at his stomach in the mirror before he eats it, wondering if it's going to affect how he looks in photos this summer. Instead he gobbles it up and then will probably come back asking for more, then you say no, so he goes and humps his poor one-eyed, abused looking teddy bear (why does no one ever buy the dog a new teddy bear?), and rolls over to go to sleep.

Dogs and other animals (to our knowledge), lack this luxury of contemplation. (Side note – I love animals, we're still animals ourselves, and, are by no means more important than any other species, we all evolved different qualities and strengths, ours just happens to be a cognitive one.)

What often happens though, is that sometimes our instincts still overpower us, disguise themselves as rational thoughts even. 'I'll eat more now because I skipped breakfast' – that's a classic instinct in disguise as a thought – your instinct tells you 'more food' and the reasoning behind it (the thought) is the disguise. Another problem we have is that our thinking brain also wants to take the lead – 'I'm not going to eat that as there's too much fat and it's not going to help me lose weight' or 'I'm skipping dinner every night this week as I have a holiday coming up.' Our thinking brain wants to do things logically. It wants order, it wants to set goals and make plans. It's the thinking brain that puts us on diets and makes us feel guilty when we give into our instincts and overindulge. When we let the thinking brain take control, we can end up doing things like undereating, overthinking, and increasing our anxiety.

So that's why sometimes it seems like there's two of us in there, playing tug of war. *The instinctive us* and *The logical us*. But I'm going to make it that bit more confusing by telling you there's not two of you, there's actually three.

The three you's
Your instincts – The instinctive you
Your thinking brain – The logical you
Your intuition – The intuitive you

So what is intuition then? Intuition is the little voice, the voice that isn't really a voice at all. It's more of an inner knowing, a feeling. For example, your instincts are telling you to eat, your thoughts are giving you reasons why you should and shouldn't, and your intuition is telling you how you actually *feel*. Your intuition is always there, it's just that sometimes we forget it or don't realise it because we're so consumed by our thoughts and urges. Thoughts can be so loud and urges can feel so strong that they often drown out our intuition, but if we take a moment to stop, quiet down the inner noise, and listen, it's there. It's *always* there. You might even say that you *are* your intuition, and your thoughts and instincts are just here to help guide you. Both your thoughts and instincts have valid points and intentions to help, but let one take too much of the lead and you become imbalanced. To make it work you just have to use your intuition to find the balance between them.

You can use your intuition in all aspects of your life, but this book, is about how to use it, with food.

TAKEAWAY

We are not our instincts and we are not our thoughts.

I allow myself quiet moments throughout the day to feel what my intuition is telling me

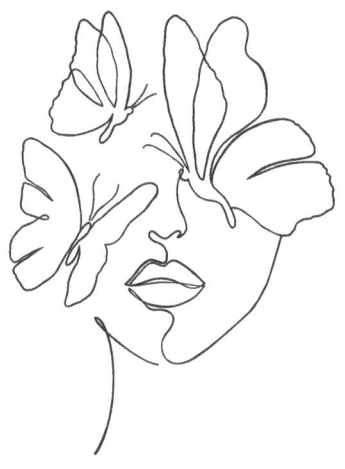

Why diets don't work

The reason why I decided to go down the path of Intuitive Eating was because I wanted to change my whole relationship with food. Food, for me anyway, is one of the most enjoyable and natural pleasures on this planet. Without sounding like too much of a hippy (it's probably already too late) but it's really amazing when you think about it. Food has been put here as a gift to us by Mother Nature, and it's remarkable the number of different recipes, cuisines, desserts and snacks we can create with such simple things that grow from the earth. I didn't want to spend the rest of my life having a bad relationship with such a natural and essential part of life. I wanted to be able to eat foods that I love and enjoy every moment of it, without feeling bad about it afterwards.

Intuitive Eating was something that in the past I had briefly heard of but didn't really understand or give much of a second thought to. I was a bit sceptical at first, but then when I started to look into it, I felt something click, like it put all of my past experiences with food and dieting into place. I realised why it felt like nothing would ever work long term for me, why I always found myself back at square one. This whole time I'd been fighting my natural urges, so I fixed on trying to control them and trying to change myself. It never even crossed my that actually I should be doing the exact opposite.

I personally didn't really ever follow set diets, it was more going through phases of eating super 'clean', having small portion sizes and not allowing myself any sugar. I thought being hungry was a good sign, that it meant I must be losing weight. The only thing is, I wasn't losing weight at all. I was constantly stuck in a cycle of eating my super 'clean' tiny portions (my 'diet') and then eventually cracking and giving up. And once you crack after depriving your body of certain foods that it's used to and loves so much, it's extremely hard to go back to your super 'healthy' ways. So, you crack once, you and crack twice, and then f*ck it. CRACK CRACK CRACK CRACK. Say crack again. And then you look back the weekend and feel ashamed of every little Lindt ball and cheesy chip you mindlessly consumed. You were at your mum's house on Sunday and she made a huge roast dinner, with homemade Yorkshire puddings and some sticky toffee pudding for dessert. It would have been rude not to eat it. Maybe the seconds weren't so necessary though. So, you beat yourself up about that too. Filled with guilt and shame, the next Monday comes, and that's it. Back to starving mode. And this time it's *really* different. Let's see how long it lasts.

For me, I was obsessed with juice cleansing. Because I would see immediate results. Got a holiday coming up? Juice cleanse. Got a wedding to attend in a few days? Juice cleanse. Need to fit into that dress but no time for the gym? Juice cleanse. There. All your problems solved. I was a juice cleanse freak, I loved it. I started with a one-day cleanse and then went to two, tried a three day and then would even try do a week at times (I usually would crack before the end though due to headaches and feeling faint). Sometimes I would even just skip dinner and have a juice instead to wake up extra skinny in the morning. There was just one problem (aside from the fact I really missed actually chewing food). It was that although I loved how I looked whilst being on the juice cleanse, the second I went back to eating normally again (healthily even), my body would return to be exactly how it was before. Another juice cleanse anyone?

The reason why you look so skinny whilst being on the cleanse is because of a lack of food in your GI tract (the GI tract is the tract from your mouth to your anus). So basically, you appear skinnier because you are completely empty inside. On top of that, the lack of protein you are consuming can cause muscle loss, which ultimately slows down the metabolism, which could actually cause potential weight gain in the future. Not only this but something happens when

you deprive yourself of calories. Your body, being the clever being it is, learns to support itself efficiently with the number of calories you give to it. So, by training your body to survive on less calories means that, when you eventually go back to eating how you usually would, it will store any 'extra' calories that it no longer needs as fat. Which also can lead to future weight gain. I hate to be the bearer of bad news guys, but there are no shortcuts here, unfortunately!

I have a friend who is always on a diet and trying to lose weight, when I asked her if she struggles with when to stop eating she responded, 'No, because I control the number of calories within my meals and snacks, so knowing when to stop eating is never a problem for me. I know it's safe for me to eat all of the food on my plate.' Each meal is carefully calculated so that by the end of the day she has eaten the exact number of calories she (and her personal trainer) believe her body should have consumed in a single day. But, because she wants to lose weight, she must consume even *less* calories than what would be considered normal for her BMI.

What is a calorie? A calorie is a unit of measurement and it's used to measure energy. Generally speaking, when we eat more calories than we burn on a regular basis then typically we will gain weight. So, by trying to eat less calories than we burn, we hope to lose weight. On paper, of course this will work. But in reality, how often do we really stick to this high maintenance and unfulfilling way of eating? Research has shown that people who are calorie counting actually tend to eat more of whatever the 'low calorie' food it is they're eating just to feel satisfied, compared to someone who is eating a meal with a high natural fat content (fatty foods have more calories, therefore are often avoided by calorie counters). Foods that are high in natural fats actually create more of a full sensation after eating (you eat less and feel full quicker). Fats are also the last to leave our digestive tract, therefore creating longer lasting satiety, meaning we stay full for much longer (foods like olive oil and avocado being at the top of the list). But most of these high caloric foods are often avoided for lower, less satiating foods.

There are a few problems with calorie counting. The first and main problem is that you are letting your mind, and your opinion of 'what is right' or 'what is normal' decide how many calories you consume. You're listening to your head only, not your body. Sometimes after a meal she will even still be hungry or not fully satisfied, but she ignores this message and waits patiently for the next meal. The next problem is that, it will only ever last for a while and she may even lose a bit of weight, but then eventually she will always slip back into her old eating habits.

Maybe she will eventually reach her target weight, but will she be able to stay on track and maintain this weight for the rest of her life using this method? Controlling and calculating every piece of food? Will she really be happy constantly restricting herself and overthinking everything she eats, feeling guilty if she fails one day and eats more calories than she should have?

Let's say you begin calorie counting. Perhaps one day your simply hungrier than you are the next (a very normal scenario). Should you deprive yourself the first day in order not to go over your target calorie intake and then the next day when you're not so hungry, overindulge due to the fear of missing out on calories that you won't allow yourself to have back in the future? The thing is, our weight is not determined by individual days or meals, everyone knows that, but rather by our lifestyle as a whole. The way we eat and how active we are on a consistent, long-term basis is where the results come from. Adding this pressure and guilt of calorie counting may feel good in the beginning as you feel more 'in control', but in the long term it's just unnecessary stress and as you will read later, restricting ourselves only makes things worse in the long term.

Instead of obsessing over the calorie numbers, I wonder if my friend ever stopped to ask herself 'Is my body *really* asking me for more calories than I need?' Has she ever listened to what her body is actually telling her? Is it her *body* telling her whether to stop or continue eating, or is it her *mind*? I'm sure my friend and I are not the only ones who've struggled with this or something of similar effect, whether it be a juice cleanse, Slimfast, keto, Weight Watchers or just counting calories. The question is, *Can you really see yourself doing this for rest of your life?* If the answer is *no*, then it's not a solution, and to put it bluntly, you're wasting your time.

Weight loss companies actually target people like us by using a false promise, telling us exactly what we want to hear. In fact, statistics show that 95% of diets fail and most people will regain their lost weight within one to five years. If the diets actually worked, then the diet industry wouldn't be making so much money from us. Part of Intuitive Eating is to contribute to removing the 'the diet culture' from our culture.

What is the diet culture? The diet culture is a system in which people believe one must be thin to be beautiful, and values beauty over health and wellbeing. The sole purpose of the diet is to lose weight (as opposed to being healthy) and the people who live by this care more about what they weigh, than how they feel. The diet culture is a cycle of misery and anxiety. You're not happy because you think you look too big, then you diet and you're not happy because you can't eat what or when you want. You get a brief thrill whenever you hit a target, but it's quickly dismissed with the anxiety of keeping the weight off, then when you gain it back, you're miserable again, and the cycle continues. By obeying the diet culture, we are living our lives through other people's validation, constantly trying to fit into the category of what is socially acceptable as opposed to what is individually needed.

A large part of the reason these diet methods don't work out is that, when you tell yourself that you're on a diet or even just saying you are

'healthy eating' you are telling yourself that this is not the *real* you. That this is a temporary you until you get to where you want to be. That the real you is a person who cannot be trusted around food, someone who wants to endlessly indulge in all kinds of unhealthy foods, someone you must constantly control. You do this by saying things like 'It was my birthday, so gave myself a break from eating healthy for a while' or 'Once I hit my target I might treat myself.' We try our hardest to control this person and don't allow ourselves any 'bad' foods at all. We speak badly about this person to ourselves 'Why have I got no self-control?', 'I'm so weak', 'I'm such a pig.' We avoid situations which we fear will bring out this person who we try so hard to hide, we even take extreme measures like skipping meals and social events all together.

Of course, we know it's never too long before this hungry, 'gluttonous' person shows themselves again, and this is what causes a 'yoyo' effect in our eating habits. Bouncing from one eating extreme to the other. Are you really this insatiable, eyes-bigger-than-their-bellied creature who wants to gorge on literally everything (edible) they lay eyes on? Is that really the *real* you? You may currently believe it is, hence why you're always on a diet, and you'll probably be reluctant to trying out some of the methods of Intuitive Eating, but persevere and what you'll find may surprise you.

On a diet we're pretending, forcing ourselves to be someone we're not. But we can only pretend for so long and we can only control things for a matter of time before we let up. Which is why finding out who the real you is, is the first step on the track to a lifetime of consistency. It's only with consistency where lasting changes are made. When you eat intuitively you'll never have to worry about dieting, fasting or counting calories again.

You're about to be make a change to the way you look at food, your entire relationship with it, and it probably goes against everything you've ever been taught or taught yourself to believe. But I need you to trust me, give it a go for a couple of weeks, see how it makes you feel and pay attention to what happens inside of you. I say a couple of weeks because, the first week may be completely different from the second, you may feel a bit all over the place, but it will level out as you rediscover what your body really wants. You need to give yourself time to get to know yourself all over again. Be sure to go into this wholeheartedly and don't be afraid to let go (no matter how odd it may feel).

TAKEAWAY

The way to a truly healthy body, is through consistency and peace of mind.

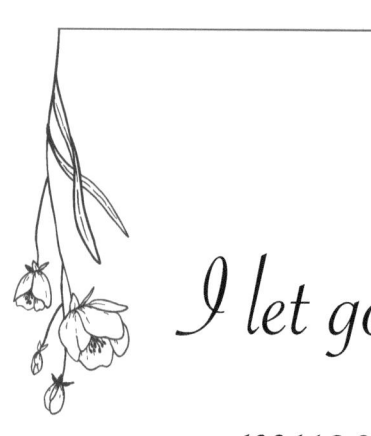

I let go of old habits and allow myself to enjoy food again.

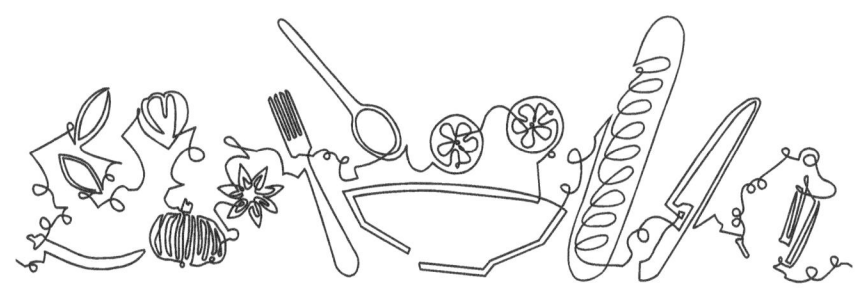

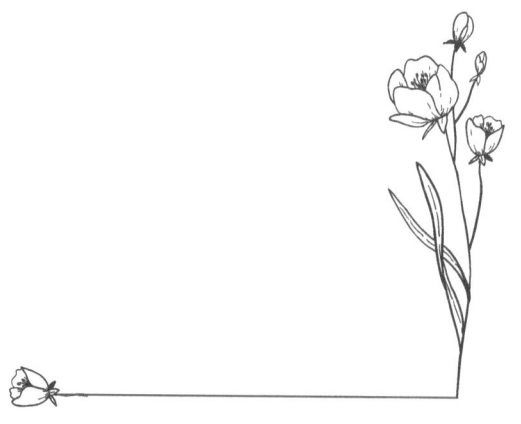

How to eat intuitively

Intuitive Eating is basically the opposite of dieting. We're no longer trying to plan, control and overthink. Instead *we feel, we listen* and *we give ourselves permission*. We work with our bodies by becoming more aware of them. No more starving them, stuffing them and then looking in the mirror stressing over them. It's not just about how we eat, but it's also how we feel about our bodies. It's about self-love and self-acceptance. We learn to enjoy food guilt-free, we no longer fear judgment from others or feel the need to be accepted because we accept ourselves. As this stress lifts off our shoulders, we become lighter and gain a more positive and confident attitude towards ourselves and the outside world. By strengthening our mind-to-body connection we learn to appreciate our bodies, putting an end to the inner battle – us vs food and our minds vs our bodies. We're now working with our bodies, eating to nourish them because, our ultimate goal, is to live a long and healthy life. And we can accomplish all this, in just two simple steps.

Step 1: Listen
Intuitive Eating tells you to listen to your body. Listen to when it's hungry and *eat*. But also, listen to when you're *full* and respect its fullness. It's basically that simple. Your body's hunger is a message, it's telling you it needs food to convert into energy to be able to support you throughout your day and to keep you and all organs, alive and healthy. Don't ignore it. Also, when you're full, don't ignore it. When you're no longer hungry, it means your body is satisfied and has had enough food to turn into energy to support you for now. Let go of the planning, controlling and judging that our minds naturally try and do, and just focus on your body, and how it feels. The best way to do this is by practicing mindful eating, which we speak about in depth in just a few pages.

Step 2: Give yourself permission
When you eat intuitively, you give yourself absolute permission to eat anything and *everything*. By giving yourself permission to eat anything you like, you are taking away the punish and reward system, e.g. 'I ate a slice of cake so I must punish myself by skipping dinner tonight.' By allowing yourself to eat whatever you want, you stop the battle in your head of what's allowed and what's not allowed, what's 'good' and what's 'bad'.

What if I told you all food was equal? You'd probably laugh in my face. 'Of course, all food is not equal! So, you mean to tell me that broccoli has the same health benefits as a bar of Carberry's Dairy Milk chocolate?!?!.' That's a rational response, and it was also my first response. Completely ridiculous right? But actually, what you eat for you next meal will neither kill you nor make you stronger. Eat one takeaway and you won't be any fatter, just as eating an apple won't make you any skinnier. However, both *will* give you sufficient energy. Eat only broccoli for the rest of your life and you'll have just as many problems as if you only ate chocolate for the rest of your life. As the saying goes – the poison is in the dose. This doesn't mean you have to ignore any current knowledge you have on foods (or refuse to learn anything new) – yes spinach is a good source of vitamins, and chocolate digestives are high in sugar – but *all* food is a chance of energy conversion. Don't let this knowledge make you label these foods as 'good' or 'bad.' It's not serving you any good. So, GIVE YOURSELF PERMISSION.

Part of the reason we crave 'bad' foods or overindulge when we eat things like chocolate or cake is because of the fact that we've put them in the 'bad' category. Just look at Eve, the forbidden fruit is always more tempting, isn't it? And this doesn't just happen with food, ever walk past a sign that says 'Do not touch'? Well I didn't really want to touch an electric fence anyway, but for some reason now I do. Or when you see a sign at the zoo that says 'Do not put your fingers in the cage.' Who on this earth needs telling not to poke their fingers into a cage with a wild animal? But now you've said it, maybe I will. And while I'm at it, I might just go fishing where the no fishing sign is, and smoking where the no smoking sign is, not that I fish or smoke, but tell me not to, and maybe I'll start. There's a famous quote – 'Try to pose yourself this task: not to think of a polar bear, and you will see that the cursed thing will come to mind every minute' (Fyodor Dostoevsky, *Winter Notes on Summer Impressions*, 1863). This theory was latter tested by a social psychologist professor at Harvard university named Daniel Wegner in 1987. He asked a group of participants to visualise their thoughts for five minutes, but told them not to think of a white bear, and if they did think of a white bear, they were to ring a bell that was placed in front of them. You can probably guess what happened next, and not only were the participants ringing the bell, but on average, they were thinking of a white bear more than once per minute! Despite the explicit instructions not to. Through performing experiments such as the white bear theory, scientists came to discover a type of psychological behaviour called reactance. Reactance occurs when a person feels that their freedom of choice is being threatened, like someone is taking away their free will, and it's this response system that's making us want to do things that we're told not to. I'm not a neuroscientist, so I won't try to delve into the depths of the mind to uncover this annoying human response that's programmed into us all. But what I do know is, the more we tell ourselves we can't have something, the more we want it. Poor Eve never really stood a chance.

This is why it's so important to give yourself permission to eat everything, because if you set certain foods as off-limits, you are theoretically, taking away your own free will. You're challenging your own mind. When you're eating a chocolate bar, sure it tastes good, but that last bite of the chocolate bar is never as good as the first. So why do we keep eating it? Because, it's the forbidden fruit. Something we're not supposed to be having so we want more of it. And besides, maybe tomorrow will be the first successful day of our never-ending diet and we won't be able to have it ever again. So we better eat as much as we can now, to really make the most of it before it's too late.

Whereas, if you see food as equal and you give yourself total permission to eat it, this chocolate bar becomes completely guilt-free and you know that there will be plenty more if it in your future, whenever you want it. Then, you might find that when you eat it, you don't actually want the entire thing. Maybe, a couple of pieces is enough for you, maybe just getting the taste is enough. If you've had a couple pieces and are still hungry, keep eating. If you're no longer hungry and do not wish to continue eating, then save the rest for later. By putting an end to the good vs bad food battle that you've got going on in your head, you're taking away all of the forbidden fruits. Therefore, eliminating the pressure of reactance towards that particular food. Only by giving yourself total permission to eat everything, can you open yourself up to discovering what you really like. What your body really wants.

Giving yourself permission to eat anything may sound like a scary, slippery slope to go down at first, because maybe you don't trust yourself. When I began my Intuitive Eating journey I (like many others) truly believed that if I gave myself the total freedom of eating whatever the hell I wanted (or thought I wanted), that I would live off of biscuits, chocolates and take outs, get ten stone heavier and develop so many health problems. But I thought, f*ck it. I've got nothing to lose trying it out and I'm sick of being stuck in this endless diet circle I've put myself in. The funny thing is, I found myself eating *less* than before. By listening to when I actually became full, I realised I'd been unconsciously overeating this whole time (or perhaps sometimes I knew I was full but would continue eating the 'bad' food through fear of not being able to eat it again). And by giving myself total permission to eat whatever I wanted, I realised I actually *wanted* the 'healthy' food I had been 'forcing' myself to eat the whole time.

Of course, in the beginning I took advantage of the 'see all food as equal' situation and I went to the local pizza takeaway store and ordered whatever I desired, guilt-free. As I ate, I listened to my body, slowed down and enjoyed the food, chewed and tasted it properly, and I found I didn't nearly eat half as much as I would have usually forced myself to eat. And I didn't feel the need to either, because, why would I? I can have another takeaway tomorrow if I like, I can even have another in a few hours when I become hungry again if I wanted. But, by the next time I noticed I was hungry (and I had it planned out, next was a Chinese followed by chocolate pudding), I didn't actually want another takeaway, or chocolate or sweets at all. Sounds like madness I know. But it's true. Nowadays, when I want a takeaway I get one, but the majority of the time I actually enjoy cooking and eating more fresh food. The only difference is, now I'm doing it because I *want* to not because I feel I have to. It's crazy how I had to first allow myself to eat whatever I wanted to be able to realise what it was I actually wanted. Just under one year later (and much to my surprise as I had been happily eating what I wanted), I realised I had actually lost a stone (6.3 kg). Losing weight was something that seemed like huge battle before, whereas now that I genuinely stopped prioritising my weight and started to relax and enjoy food, it seemed to be falling off me.

TAKEAWAY

> *Feel, listen and give yourself permission. Whenever we tell ourselves we can't have something, we want it more. Only when we let go of this habit can we discover what we really want.*

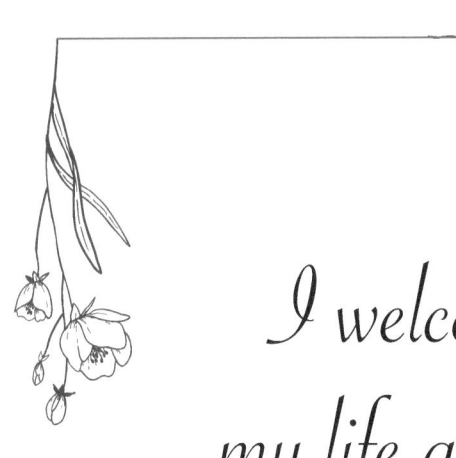

I welcome all foods into
my life and I eat them with
great pleasure.

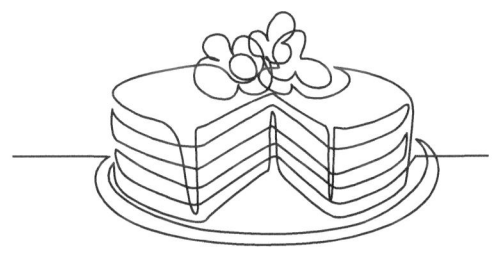

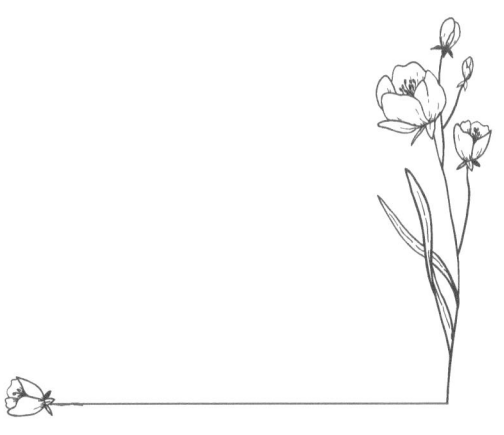

Respecting your fullness

There will be times when you feel the urge to continue eating even when you're full. The trick is to become aware of yourself doing this, whether it's in the moment of temptation or a whole bag of chocolate covered Oreos later (whoops). But as long as at some point you become aware of yourself slipping back into those old habits, that's the first step back on track. Eventually, the goal is, to be aware of yourself *all* the time and mindless eating will be a thing of the past. It's important to remember that there's always a reason for everything, there's even a reason you feel the need to continue eating when you're no longer hungry, and let's look at some of them…

'You have to finish your plate' –

This is a common phrase I'm sure most of us have heard at some point. When I was a child I wasn't allowed to leave the table until my plate was finished. 'There are people in Africa starving' as my mum or dad would say. So even though sometimes you're completely full halfway through dinner, you plough through, gnawing your way to the finish line, because, well, that's the right thing to do, right? You don't want to waste the food after all. Well intuitive eating say's it's ok to stop halfway through a meal, *if* you feel full (or have another plate *if* you're still hungry). If you don't want to waste

food (I hate to waste food) then wrap it up and put it in the fridge for later or the next day even (leftovers taste better anyways). Yes, it is terrible that there are people starving in the world and there are so many charities you can sign up to if you want to help. But if you've had enough, and that bowl of pasta just isn't as appealing as it once was, it's not doing anyone any good by forcing it down. Not you. Not Africa. After a while of listening to your body you'll get to know yourself and find it much easier for you to adjust your portion sizes accordingly.

You're enjoying the taste of the food and you don't want it to end –

Ok this is the one for me, the one I can say I struggled with the most. When you're halfway through indulging in that homemade sticky toffee pudding and then it comes over you, you're full. And you know it. Well, the good news is that you know it, you're listening to your body, yay. But now where do you find the strength to do as your body's telling you and stop eating? Willpower comes into play a bit here (I'd be lying if I said it didn't). Meditation also helps *a lot* with this (meditation in general I mean, you don't have to be meditating while eating, duh). But once you've become aware of the fact that your body is beginning to feel satiated and you're no longer hungry, let that be a signal to at least slow down. Take a moment, to breathe, listen to your stomach (your food isn't going anywhere) and give yourself *total* permission to continue. Remind yourself that there will be much more food in the future for you to enjoy whenever you please. There's no right or wrong choice here, you absolutely can finish every last bite if you want to, completely guilt-free. Just be sure to eat every bite slowly and mindfully, and enjoy it. As we pay closer attention while we're eating, we usually notice that, past a certain point the food stops tasting as good. Generally, the less hungry we are the less were actually enjoying the taste. In fact, often what we're doing when we continue to eat for this reason, is we're holding onto the memory of what the first bite tasted like. However, if we stop and take notice, we would likely find that it's really not tasting the same as this stage.

You're bored –

I think after the year 2020–2021 we can all relate to this one. The urge to boredom eat definitely came over me more than a few times during the lockdowns of 2020. The first step in dealing with this is to take the time to listen to what your body is telling you, maybe you actually are hungry. If so, eat. But if you know you're not hungry and are just looking for something to fill the time, consider some other things you can do with this time instead of eating. Remember, you are *bored* not hungry. There are so many perhaps even more enjoyable and productive activities you could do. To name a few: journaling (you would be surprised how much you get into

this and it's really quite therapeutic), drawing, painting, sport, reading, meditating, playing a game, etc. The list goes on. Find something that works for you and next time you feel the urge to boredom eat, occupy your mind with one of these tasks and see how it goes.

Wanting a specific taste –

The first thing to note here is that, the fact that you are thinking about food may be because you are actually hungry. If so, you know what to do. However, it is also possible that you are not hungry and you just really enjoy the flavour of a particular food. If this is the case, don't tell yourself you can't have something, as it will only make you want it more (forbidden fruit). Instead, let yourself have the food. When you eat it, make sure you really enjoy it. Focus on what you're eating, the flavours, the textures, sensations it gives you. For me, chocolate is my weakness and I used to struggle with the problem of craving the taste and then going too far and consuming the entire bar, when I really didn't even want the whole thing. You crave the taste and then once you begin eating the food, mindless eating takes over. Now when I crave chocolate (which is often) I give myself total permission to eat it instead of trying to tell myself no, I enjoy it SO much more and I eat a hell of a lot less of it. And what's even better, I still feel great after, no shame, no guilt.

You're a 'sugar addict' –

I don't know who needs to hear this but, let's just get one thing straight, YOU ARE NOT A SUGAR ADDICT. Please stop telling yourself that mantra. It's only making you believe it's true. If a drug addict for example, would be sitting in a room with a pile of drugs on the table in front of them, they wouldn't care what they had to do to get their fix, inhale, inject, eat it (or insert into other orifices). They would be craving it so much they'd be willing to consume it in any way shape or form. If you were in a room, and a pile of plain white granulated sugar was on the table in front of you, I highly doubt you would be tempted to eat it, let alone consume it in any of the other options above. You are not addicted to sugar, you enjoy the taste of certain foods with sugar in, but you are not addicted to the sugar itself. Don't mistake desire for addiction. Consider the possibility that the reason you feel like you're craving sugar is because you are telling yourself you cannot, or should not, be eating it. Likewise, if we (suddenly) deprive ourselves of something, it can make our want for that specific thing much stronger.

Emotional eating –
Many of us are guilty of doing this at some point. Your partner just broke up with you and all you want to do is curl up on the sofa with a huge jar of Nutella and watch the notebook. Or maybe you're stressed about something and you find yourself snacking more often as a way to distract yourself. We find things like food and drinks comforting because they give us instant pleasure and they make us feel good, but you should always remember that it is only temporary. And once it's over, you will go back to feeling the same way you did

before. Emotional eating is not resolving any of your current issues, so why then add the problem of overeating on top of what you're already dealing with? The best thing to do in this situation is to allow yourself to feel your emotions. Instead of looking for a way out, a quick fix, turn and face your problems head on and embrace them, let yourself cry if that's what you feel you need to do. Crying has been shown to reduce stress and it actually releases endorphins (the happy chemical) in the brain. Not the same as Nutella for example, which releases dopamine (the want chemical, as we will talk about more later). It's only once you allow yourself to embrace your emotions that you can fully begin to move on and find solutions. The best way to do this, is through meditation, as when we meditate we observe our thoughts and feelings, allowing ourselves to feel them but not to get attached to them. To observe them, through a non-judgmental point of view. That being said, if you've taken the time to embrace your emotions and still all you want is something edible to comfort yourself with, then please, give yourself permission and allow yourself to enjoy it as much as possible, without regrets. It's no secret that food can make us feel good and it's not a crime to use it for that, just eat mindfully so you don't pass the point of feeling good.

Eating out of habit –
This maybe your daily stop at Starbucks in the morning before you get to the office, one full fat iced latte and a blueberry muffin, standard. Maybe you always have your

afternoon snack at 4 pm. Or maybe you're ordering a burger and you just get the fries because what psycho orders a burger with no fries? The trick here is to really be aware of how you're feeling during these habits. How much are you enjoying that Starbucks in the morning? Do you really enjoy it or are you just passing time before you get to the office? Are you actually hungry at 4 pm or eating out of habit? Do you really want the fries or are you ordering them just because they come with the meal?

Eating for the occasion –
This includes birthdays, weddings, Christmas and pretty much any event that involves food. Remember that just because it's a special occasion it doesn't mean you have to eat any differently as you normally would, treat it as any other day (foodwise) and give yourself complete permission to eat whatever you want. Don't feel bad about eating the birthday cake, but at the same time don't feel the need to over indulge *just* because it's a birthday.

Mindless eating –
This is a sticky one because – hence the name – half the time when we're doing it, we don't realise it. We're watching a movie and we are downing the popcorn like there's no tomorrow, so engrossed in the film that we don't even stop to look at it until we've hit the bottom of the bag. Munching on a bag of M&Ms whilst on the phone to your friend, chatting away and your hand is working on autopilot just bringing the food to your mouth. The way to avoid doing this sounds pretty obvious, it's to eat mindfully. But actually, the hard part (not so hard once you get the hang of it) is to catch yourself in the act. It's like we said with the chocolate covered Oreos, as long as at some point you catch yourself (even if it's after it's happened), you're doing something right. Maybe next time you will catch yourself during the act, then, eventually before it even happens. It's the becoming aware that is important here. Practicing the mindful eating exercise in this book is the best way to do this. Eventually, the more you practise, it will become like a second nature to you.

Understanding the reasons why you're wanting to continue eating even though you're not hungry is important. It's important because once you're aware of something, you then can choose how to respond to it. And it's the response which makes all the difference.

Sure, there will be times you'll maybe drift back into your old ways of over (or under) indulging, which is completely normal. Old habits don't often die so easily. So don't be so hard on yourself when this happens, forgive yourself. You're human and it's totally normal. I still have days where I slip up and overindulge when my body really didn't want it (more so in the beginning of my journey, due to Intuitive Eating these moments are far and few between now), then I naturally would begin to feel ashamed of what I had eaten, and become tempted to continue acting out old habits, because that's just what I was used to doing for so long previously. But by totally forgiving yourself you make peace with any mistakes you feel you made. You acknowledge you may have slipped up and eaten more than a comfortable amount, and you remind yourself that you're human, it happens and it's part of the journey. Just like in meditation, be sure to bring your attention back to the present and stop thinking and worrying about what has already happened.

TAKEAWAY

Becoming aware of our current habits will give us the opportunity to make conscious decisions.

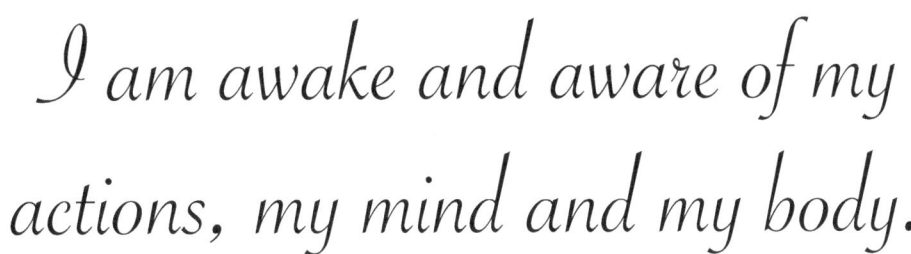

I am awake and aware of my
actions, my mind and my body.

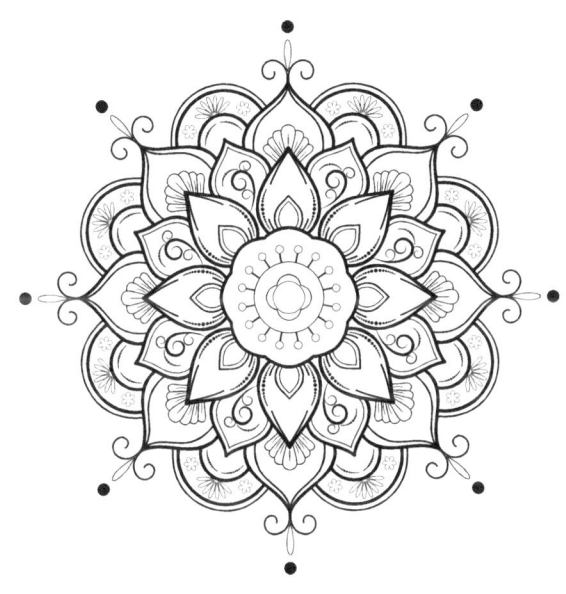

The importance of self-forgiveness

Self-forgiveness plays a key role in Intuitive Eating. Think of it like this, you've had an argument with a friend. Could you move on with your friendship without truly forgiving one another? Maybe you do stay friends, but because you were not able to forgive each other, more arguments are bound to keep arising in the future. It's because by not forgiving you're holding on to any negative emotions toward that person (whether it be conscious or unconscious). Maybe you've forgotten what the argument was even about. But you remember the feelings you hold toward this person and this is what causes future problems. It's the same with food. If you beat yourself up over something you've eaten and don't forgive yourself, it allows the negative feelings you are holding to be attached to that food you've just eaten, which then places that food into the 'bad category' (which should no longer exist). This then encourages the punish/reward system next time you eat that particular food and sets you up for more of these bingeing experiences and guilty feelings in the future.

But by forgiving yourself you take away all of those shameful, regretful, guilty feelings and reduce the chance of any self-sabotaging thoughts and acts going forward. The best thing you can do at this moment is to accept what has happened, show yourself some compassion and to look forward with a clear, non-judgmental, more positive head on your shoulders. Forgiving yourself may be difficult at first as it's not what you're used to doing and it takes strength, but at the same time, it's the most natural and pleasant thing you can do, and it is the key to determining how you will act in the future.

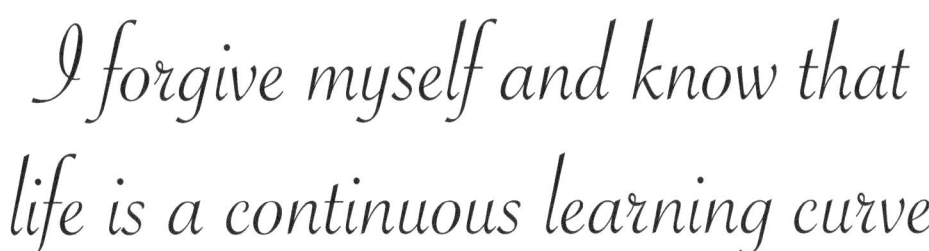

I forgive myself and know that
life is a continuous learning curve

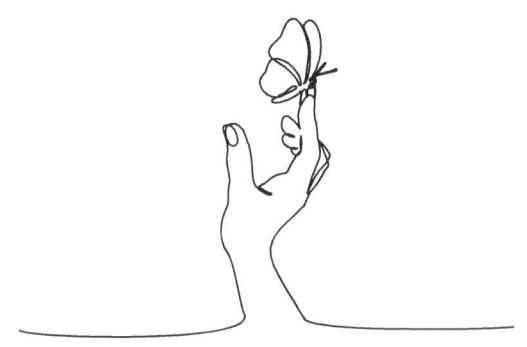

Chasing the reward

It's helpful to fill your fridge and cupboards with as much fresh food as possible, this way you are naturally more inclined to eat this type of food. Whilst as an Intuitive Eater we see all food as equal, we must understand that some types of food are simply harder for us to stop eating once we're satiated than others are. These are generally foods high in sugar and foods that have been processed, and big food companies know exactly how to make them even more irresistible to us. Did you know that it's literally someone's job to sit there and taste food to rate how addictive it is? These 'craving experts', let's call them, will trial foods to find the exact level which the human tastebuds are experiencing the maximum amount of pleasure. They call this the 'bliss point'. It allows them to capture the perfect amount of salt, sugar and fat to activate our taste buds to just the right level which will leave us wanting more. And this is the reason why we find many processed foods harder to stop eating; they're engineered to set off to the reward system in our brain and make us want more. As we eat these foods they release a chemical in our brains called dopamine (aka: *the want chemical*), and the next time we see that food, our brains will remember and will already start producing dopamine just from looking at it. In this scenario it's much easier for us to lose control and overindulge. The dopamine is telling us we want more, to keep chasing the reward, even when our bodies are not hungry. Whilst we are not actually addicted to these foods we are certainly more tempted by them than we are to other more whole and natural foods. For example, how many times have you found yourself uncontrollably eating apples? Or pears? Or broccoli? That's because nature isn't trying to trick you into eating more than you need. The temptation of the promise of reward. But that's all dopamine is, a *promise* of reward, not the reward itself. The majority of the time, the wanting sensation is stronger than the actual pleasure of the reward itself. Just think about anytime you've eaten something high in sugar or salt, how much are you really enjoying the last bite? Probably not even one-tenth as much as you enjoyed the first. But you continue, because the dopamine in your brain is telling you to chase the reward. This neurotransmitter really doesn't mean bad at all, it actually helps us in much more ways than harms us. Imagine it didn't exist, we would either die from starvation due to not wanting any food, or we'd become extinct from a lack of attraction to the opposite sex, or best-case scenario, we'd survive, but be a bunch of underachievers with very little motivation in life. It's just unfortunate that big food companies have figured out how to use these important brain chemicals against us for their own benefits.

When these dopamine inducing foods are around us, they can make the other foods seem somewhat invisible. For example, you're less likely to eat a piece of fruit if there's a Snickers bar around, because, although fruit tastes just as amazing, it only releases the 'right' amount of dopamine into your system, enough for you to know you want the fruit and you enjoy eating it, but you're also more aware of when to stop eating. Rather than a doctored chocolate bar that tricks your brain into thinking your body wants more than it actually does. When we eat more natural foods, we find it easier to listen to what our body's and give them what they need, rather than making decisions hyped up on dopamine. If you want to eat these foods, which we all do from time to time, then by all means, allow yourself to eat them. Just remember to eat them slowly be extra mindful so you can really know when you're satiated. It's important to stop seeing these foods as 'bad' because the truth is, a little of this food isn't bad at all, you can eat these foods and still live a long healthy life. When I look at people like my 96-year-old grandad who lived in an apartment in the UK on his own, fit and healthy most of his life. I've seen him eat cake, dessert, lasagnes and pasta (almost every day the pasta). But I also noticed a couple of other things about him. The first is that, I've never seen him eat to the point where he complains he's *too* full. The second is that, he takes his time, I've never in my life seen him gobble something up quickly, he's never 'stuffing his face,' usually he's the last at the table to finish.

So many people on diets try and cut out all the 'bad' food completely and the truth is, not only does it suck the fun out of eating and set you up for future relapses, but it's just not necessary. Food is here to nourish our bodies and give us energy, but also for us to enjoy (or else it wouldn't taste so good). That also means not eating past the point of enjoyment, otherwise what's the point? Our bodies don't need it, and we're no longer enjoying it, we're only continuing because we're chasing a reward that's been and gone.

A good way to understand if you really want to continue eating or to eat something at all is to wait ten minutes. Sometimes, if I've had a snack, and I think I want another, I simply give myself permission to do so but agree to wait ten minutes to see if I still want it then. Most of the time, after the ten minutes is up, I've realised I'm satisfied with what I had eaten and no longer want to eat more. The reason this happens is because immediately after we've eaten, dopamine, the want chemical, is still fired up and running through our brains, but if you wait a few minutes, the temptation (the dopamine) usually calms down and our brains connect with our stomachs to realise just how satiated we actually are.

TAKEAWAY

Surround yourself with nourishing whole foods.

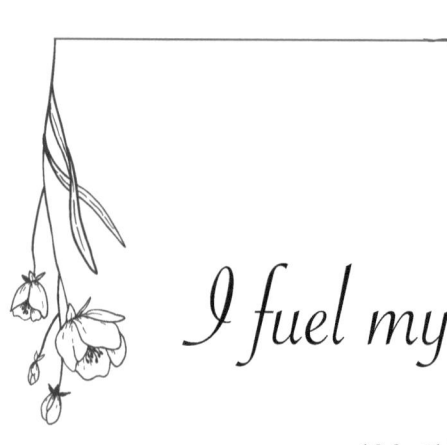

I fuel my body with foods that make me feel good

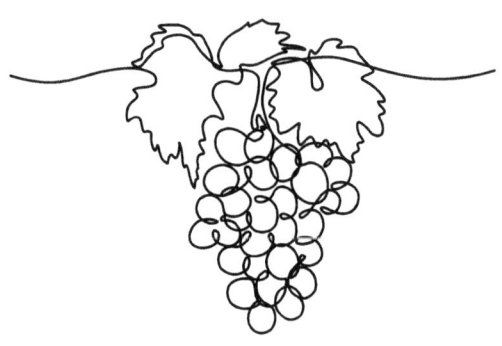

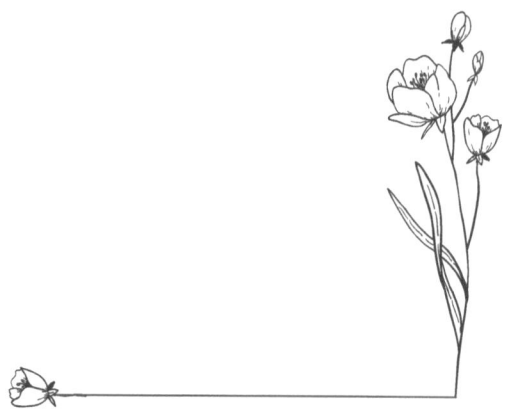

Meditation

Meditation helps for so many reasons when it comes to Intuitive Eating and it's really an essential part of it. When we meditate, we are repetitively bringing our attention back to focusing on one thing, usually our breath. It can be tiring and, in the beginning, even a little frustrating. But ultimately, it's great training for the brain. To be honest, it helps in *all* aspects of your life, and it's very transformative. But let's take a look at how exactly it can help you to eat intuitively.

One of the things that the specific action of repetitively redirecting our attention to one thing teaches us, which helps a great deal with Intuitive Eating, is patience. Patience helps us to be able to slow down and take necessary pauses when we are eating, even when we have the urge to eat fast. But this act of patience is so much more than simply eating slowly. When we use patience what we're doing is delaying instant gratification for a more valued reward in the future (in this case our health). Using patience to go against our natural urge to eat fast also means using willpower, and having self-control. Something many people wish they had more of but are unsure how to attain. By practicing Intuitive Eating, we strengthen our willpower every day, and the benefits of this reach out

far beyond our dinner tables. It affects our entire lives. How we do one thing is often an example of how we do all things, so if we have more willpower when eating then we also have more willpower for things like exercise, our jobs, changing our habits and achieving our goals.

Along with patience, meditation teaches us calmness, and when we are calm we live in a more peaceful headspace, a more stress-free headspace (reducing stress is usually the reason people get into meditation in the first place). By reducing stress, we become happier people on the whole. I always heard the rumours of this, but somehow, I was still pleasantly surprised when I began feeling these effects on myself. I would find myself smiling more for no reason (sometimes I'd have to laugh at myself because what weirdo walks around smiling for no reason), petty arguments stopped bothering me and any negative feelings that I had before seemed like they were dissolving away and becoming so much less important. How does being a happier person affect our eating? It's very simple, why do people comfort eat? It's the same reason people take drugs, gamble, or go on shopping sprees with money they don't really have. To make themselves feel good. To achieve a fast high in the hope of distracting themselves from how they really feel. These people are not happy so they search for happiness externally. But a truly happy person doesn't need these external influences to make themselves feel good, because their happiness is already coming from the inside. Practicing regular meditation gives you this inner happiness, and with it, things like comfort eating will become a thing of the past.

Just because your mind is calm however, doesn't mean that you will turn into this super-chilled hippy, just relaxing and smiling all day. In fact, the opposite will happen. Because you'll be using so much less energy for all the overthinking, worrying and everything else that you used to stress over, you'll have even more energy for things like working out and being motivated in other areas of your life. Calm and happy people have *more* energy. They also forgive more easily too. So next time you feel you ate a bit more than what your body needed, or a type of food you'd normally feel guilty over, with a calm and positive mind, you'll find it much easier to forgive yourself and move on.

This calm mind will also enable us to sleep better (I personally began meditating for that exact reason). I found that when I slept well and was less tired in the day, I had less cravings for fast energy releasing foods like sugary snacks and refined carbs. Having more energy from a good night's sleep replaced the need to look to food to boost my energy levels. Research has shown that sleep deprivation actually causes an increase in overall hunger. This is because when we're tired we produce higher levels of cortisol (the stress hormone), a chemical which has been proven to increase appetite. So focusing on becoming less stressed and happier should not be underestimated, it actually has an enormous effect on our relationship with food. And a sure pass to a more stress-free mind, is of course, mediation.

Sitting and spending time within ourselves teaches us mental and body awareness which allows us to do two things. The first, is to be more conscious of our thoughts. When we're more conscious of what's running through our heads we are less likely to eat mindlessly. When we feel we're losing focus on what we're eating and we're on the verge of mindless eating, then just like how we redirect our attention in meditation, we remember to bring our minds back to the present moment again and focus on the food and our body more often. Remaining in the present whilst eating makes the whole experience so much more satisfying as it allows us to enjoy the food much more and we are also much less likely to over eat as our minds are fully aware of what our bodies are telling us. The second thing is that as our body awareness grows, so does our appreciation for it. When we stop and listen to our stomachs, or focus on the feeling of our breath entering and leaving our lungs, we can't help but be more aware of the inner workings of our body's. They are constantly working, 24/7. Even when we are sleeping, they're working. It makes it easy for our intentions to shift from just wanting to fit into our pants, to wanting to be a healthier person when we genuinely appreciate and care for our bodies.

As we sit in the silence, focusing on our breath, simply noticing any bodily feelings or sounds, watching our thoughts go by without judgment, something wonderful happens inside of us. We start to become aware of the fact that we're separate from our body, not only our body but also our thoughts as well. The fact that we're observing them implies that we are not them, we are the ones who are watching and noticing them. It's a peculiar feeling but on the other hand, somewhat freeing. Meditation is life-changing because once we achieve this realisation we automatically begin to act differently. You'll think back to how much time you actually spent living in this web of thoughts and acting in line with the persona that you had created, comparing it to how you're now able to (and even perhaps automatically) just let all of the thoughts and personal judgments pass through. This separateness we feel from our thoughts makes it so much easier to let go of the negative ones and focus on the positive uplifting ones. Some more advanced meditators even choose not to become attached to any thoughts at all, negative or positive, and just simply live in the present as much as possible. We're not our thoughts, so just because one arises, it does not mean we need to get caught up in it. Instead, we simply observe it from a neutral perspective,

allowing it to be there and allowing it to pass, just as we do in the practice of meditation itself. The separateness we feel towards our body is in no way a feeling of disconnection. We feel more connected to our body than ever before because we are now so much more aware of them. However, it does makes us feel more inclined to treat our body almost as if it were a separate person, someone we really care for. We want this person, who we use to manoeuvre through life performing all of our daily tasks, communicating our thoughts with the outside world, to be strong and healthy. We want the best for them so we treat them with respect and love. We naturally will feel more inclined to do this by eating nourishing foods, respecting our fullness and staying active.

Following the daily meditation exercise in this book every day is enough to provide you with all of the benefits above. When you think of the amount of time we all spend on social media, watching Netflix or messaging our friends in group chats, things which are usually pretty unproductive, 20 minutes a day to completely transform your mind and body, is really nothing. If it's your first time meditating and in the beginning you feel impatient or like it's not working, I urge you to stick to it. This feeling is completely normal and with more practise it will begin to feel more natural, although in the beginning you may feel like you have to push yourself to stick with it, the more you begin feeling the benefits, the more you will find you want to do it. Please remember, every day our thought activity is different, some days our minds will be racing and other times they will be calmer. Our hormones also fluctuate, and the amount of sleep we've had the previous night is sometimes different, affecting our mood and how tired we feel. All these factors amongst many others come into play when determining how active our minds will be and how easy we will find it to stay focussed when meditating. But the one thing we can be sure of is that the more often and consistently we practice, the more relaxed, happier and focused we will be on the whole, body and mind.

TAKEAWAY

Meditating regularly will have a profound impact on your mind and body.

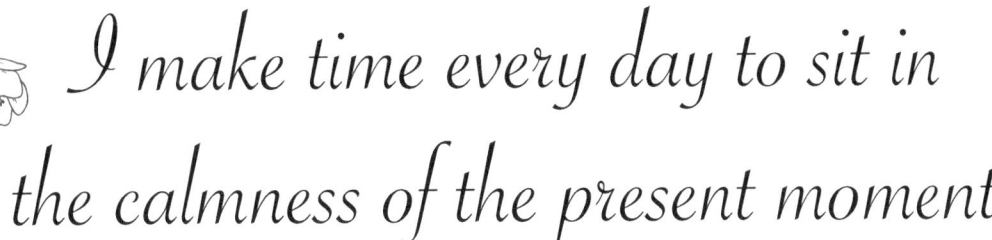

I make time every day to sit in the calmness of the present moment

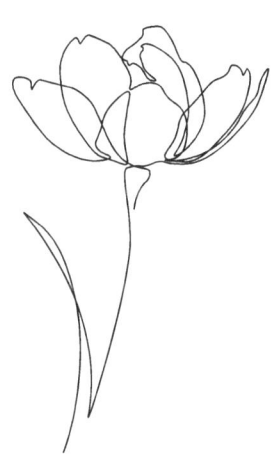

Daily meditation

Set aside time in your day especially for this one exercise.

Ideally you should do 10–20 minutes, twice a day (i.e. 10 minutes in the morning and 10 minutes in the evening). If 10–20 minutes feels too long at first, and you feel it's too difficult then you might want to start with 5 minutes and work your way up. Also feel free to do longer, but it should be no more than 30 minutes per sitting. Whatever you decide to do, make a habit of doing it every day, preferably twice a day. (If you have super busy day which we all do sometimes then at least make time to do it once.) But bear in mind, it's something that the more you do, the more you will feel the benefits. I began doing 5 minutes twice a day and I now currently do 10–20 minutes twice a day (depending on how I feel).

1. Find a comfortable spot to sit, this can be sitting on a pillow on the floor with your legs crossed or, sitting on a chair – the back should be upright, not straining but not slouching either, just relaxed whilst maintaining good posture. It's better not to lie down as you're more likely to fall asleep.

2. Either close your eyes, or if you prefer your eyes open, find a spot to hold your gaze on (it should be a low gaze, about a foot in front of you) and relax your focus.

3. Relax, and begin to notice your breath.

4. Find one particular spot you would like to focus on throughout the meditation practice. This could be the septum in your nose, the space between your nose and your top lip, the rise and fall of your chest or simply the vibrations you feel inside your nose when inhaling and exhaling.

5. Hold your focus on the chosen focus point, noticing and being aware of the breath from the very start of the inhale, to the end of the exhale and hold the focus throughout the space in-between breaths.

6. Every time a thought comes into your head, simply notice it from a non-judgmental perspective and then return your attention to the focus point.

—————————— TIP ——————————

Don't get frustrated or annoyed when thoughts come into your head, they are part of the exercise!

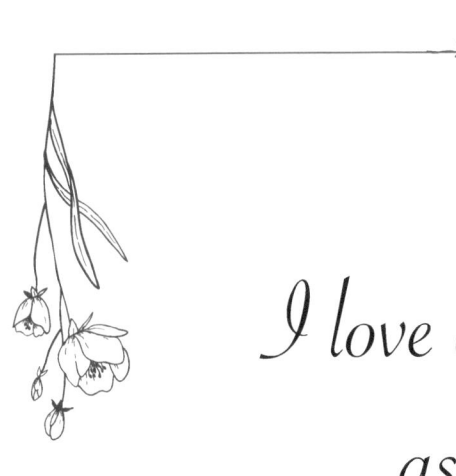

I love and accept myself

as I am today

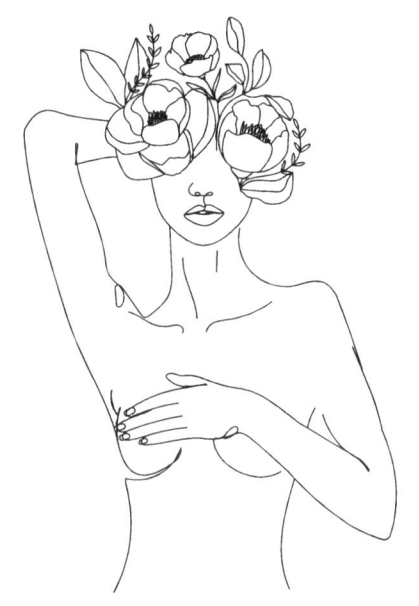

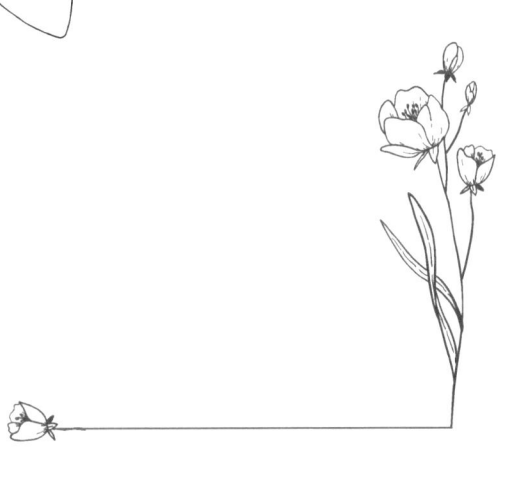

Tips for Intuitive Eating

1. Rate your hunger

A good tip when Intuitive Eating is to rate your hunger out of 8. This helps you to really be able to understand if you are hungry and just exactly how hungry you are. You can do this whenever you like throughout the day, but I recommend always checking in at these specific times: before meals, during meals, after meals, when you're wanting to snack and whilst snacking.

Below I have made a guide for you, this is the scale I use to rate my hunger, with 0–1 being not hungry at all, and 8 being starving.

Hunger Level	Current Feeling	Action to Take
Hunger Level 0–1	Not hungry at all. Full (could be after a meal when you're feeling full.)	No action to take towards eating food. If you're currently eating, consider stopping.
Hunger Level 2	Content. Not full but not hungry either.	No action to take towards eating food.
Hunger Level 3	Hunger approaches. Thoughts of food come but not necessarily wanting to eat (could take it or leave it attitude).	Simply take note that hunger is approaching. A good time to start cooking/preparing a meal if it takes a while.
Hunger Level 4	Mild hunger. Could eat but could also wait.	If you chose to eat 'little and often' now is a good time to eat.
Hunger Level 5	Hungry. Ready to eat. You feel stomach beginning to churn slightly.	Ideal meal time.

Hunger Level	Current Feeling	Action to Take
Hunger Level 6	Still hungry but your belly is rumbling a lot more. Fantasising about food.	Meal time. Be mindful not to eat too fast.
Hunger Level 7	Very hungry. Food that you wouldn't normally eat are looking a lot more appealing. Can't stop thinking about food. Losing focus on things.	Try to eat as soon as possible. Be extra mindful when eating.
Hunger Level 8	Starving mode. In pain from hunger. Feeling faint. Can't concentrate. Will eat anything at this point.	Hopefully you would never get to this point of hunger (especially if you're Intuitive Eating). But if you do, try to eat as soon as possible. Be extra mindful when eating as you are more likely to overeat.

Something that helps me a lot whenever I am tempted to continue eating past the point of hunger is, once I've rated my hunger level, saying something out loud (you can also say it 'out loud' in your head by actually speaking the words in your mind). For example, you're eating a bag of chips and you check in with your stomach and realise your hunger level is at 1, say the words 'I'm no longer hungry' either in your head or actually say it out loud (if you're alone). By doing this you're fully recognising that you no longer need to eat anymore to fuel your body and the choice you make to continue eating past this point is no longer necessary. Be sure to always give yourself total permission to continue eating if you want to, even when you're completely full.

2. Rate your fullness

I also like to rate my fullness on a scale of 1–8. This comes in handy for knowing how much food is enough for you and knowing when to stop eating. There's no right or wrong answer here, because we all have different eating habits, but by becoming aware of how full we actually are and knowing how full we want to be, it gives us more of an idea as to knowing when we want to stop eating. Someone who eats three times a day (like myself) may decide to eat to a higher fullness level of 5, than someone who eats more 'little and often' throughout the day, who might decide to stay on a more consistent level of 4. When you've reached the fullness that you're happy with, simply become aware of how you feel, be sure to never tell yourself you have to stop eating. It's also possible to feel different levels of hunger and fullness at the same time, which is why it's good to rate both. For example, just because your stomach is at a fullness level of 0 it doesn't necessarily mean that you are hungry. You can have an empty stomach and still not feel like eating and you can be somewhat full but still feel hunger. Always remind yourself that you're free to continue eating to your heart's content. I've created this as a rough guide, something that I personally use, feel free to use this or change it to your liking.

Fullness Level	Current Feeling	Action to Take
Fullness Level 0–1	Stomach feels completely empty.	If your stomach is empty and hunger arises then eat.
Fullness Level 2	Stomach feels mutual, not much feeling.	No actions to take.
Fullness Level 3	A light full feeling.	Notice the feeling. If you are eating and still hungry then continue, maybe chose to slow down at this stage.
Fullness Level 4	Full feeling comes slightly stronger, still feeling comfortable.	Slow down eating and consider to stop or take a break. Our ability to notice exactly how full we are is always delayed (as we will speak more about later), so a pause from eating at this stage could help us realise how full we really are.
Fullness Level 5	Stomach is feeling full and content.	Allow yourself to acknowledge this feeling. Consider to stop eating or at least pause.
Fullness Level 6	Full and content. Feels closer to the limit.	Listen to and respect your bodies signals. Give yourself permission to continue if you want to. Remind yourself that you can eat whatever you want in the future.

Fullness Level	Current Feeling	Action to Take
Fullness Level 7	Stomach is beginning to feel stretched.	Listen to and respect your body's signals. Give yourself permission to continue if you want to. Remind yourself that you can eat whatever you want in the future.
Fullness Level 8	About to explode. Feeling tired and sluggish. Uncomfortable. Feels sick.	At this point it's hard not to listen to what your body is telling you. Be sure to forgive yourself, this can happen to anyone from time to time and it does not affect you, your weight or your health in the grand scheme of things.

3. Don't let yourself get too hungry

When we get too hungry (say for example a hunger level of 6 or upwards) we make different food choices to what we would when we're not as hungry (like a 4 or 5). This happens because when we're hungry, our brains are essentially starved of glucose. Glucose is the main fuel for our brains, so when we're lacking it, foods that our bodies can turn into glucose faster become more appealing to us. 'Carby' and sugary foods being the fastest options. And the hungrier we get, the more appealing these foods are to us. This is why when we're really hungry it feels like we feel like we have less control over our food choices, how much and how fast we eat, and we are more attracted to foods like chocolate and pizza. Which of course, you are free to eat whatever you want, but you should try and make food choices with a clear mind, not a glucose-deprived mind. What also happens when we're in this state, is our ability to control our emotions is reduced. We can become snappy and irritable (aka 'hangry') and we lack in the ability to concentrate (your body is more focused on trying to get your attention on finding some food!). So, it's best to eat between the hunger levels of 4 and 5 whenever it's possible. This way you reduce the temptation of gobbling your food down too quickly and over eating.

4. Don't watch the scales

By using our intuition, we allow ourselves to be guided by our senses, we *feel* our way. As opposed to adding up numbers or starring at the scale. If you, like many others have spent a great deal of your life starring at the scales and measuring your waist size and are still not happy with yourself. Then let that be a sign to stop, and try a different approach.

I was once someone who was obsessed with weighing myself. So many times, I would stand on those scales and stare down at my weight, letting the number I saw determine my mood and my actions for the day ahead. Once I started Intuitive Eating I decided to stop weighing myself. Weighing only adds stress and pressure, encouraging the starving and binging cycle. I threw out any scales I had and I didn't weigh myself for nine months. It was only when I went to visit family, I saw some scales on their bathroom floor and curiosity got the better of me. I stepped onto them, and saw that I had lost weight. I couldn't believe it because for years I had been weighing myself and setting target weights to reach, only to see little to no progress. I knew I looked good and I was happy with my figure but I could never really tell if this was due to my change of mindset and the fact that I was accepting myself more, but to see an actual change in my weight confirmed it. Not only was I feeling great but I was actually making physical changes. Going forward I continue still to this this day not weighing myself. If once in a while I come across the opportunity to check my weight, and I feel like it, then I might do so. But I'm generally not bothered as I know now that knowing my weight doesn't affect my weight. Not for the better anyway.

Don't watch the scales. Don't measure yourself. Make your next move based on how you feel, *intuitively*.

5. Stay consistent with mediation

As we spoke about earlier, meditation is such an important element when Intuitive Eating. The key to really reaping the benefits of it is to stay consistent. When you start to let it slip, skip days, or let the busyness of your life take over, you'll soon begin to realise that all those benefits will also be slipping away. If you accidently miss a day once in a while it won't make much difference at all, but to maintain that tranquil state of mind you must stay consistent with it. A good way to do this is to meditate at a particular time. For example, after you wake up, after a workout, or before you go to bed. In the daily meditation exercise it says to meditate twice a day, which is ideal, but if your routine is different one day and you can't meditate at your usual time, then try to find a spare 10–20 minutes somewhere else in your day to fit it in, even if it means only meditating once instead of twice. However, this should be an exception and not a habit. Get into the routine of meditating every day, twice a day.

Mindful eating

Mindful eating is the secret weapon of Intuitive Eating. When you eat mindfully not only do you gain awareness and control over your eating habits, but you appreciate the food and you enjoy it like never before. It's also excellent brain training as it's considered a form of meditation. In fact, there are meditation retreats where people go just for this!

To become a mindful eater, you must first understand what mind*less* eating is. This way you will be able to identify just exactly how mindless/mindful you currently are.

A mindless eater is basically concentrating on anything but the food. If you're eating a sandwich on your lunch break but thinking about work related problems – you're mindless eating. If you're munching on some chocolate digestives whilst working on your school essay – you're mindless eating. If you're eating a Weight Watchers' noodle salad whilst worrying about what dress you're going to wear on Saturday night, guess what – you're mindless eating. A mindless eater eats 'on the go', multitasks and doesn't make time for food. You can be a person that knows exactly how many calories and macro/micronutrients are in your meals, but if while you're eating that meal you're not paying attention to it, then you too are a mindless eater.

Ok, so now you have an idea what exactly a mindless eater is, think about how many of those situations or something similar you've been in. Ask yourself how often you think you mindless eat. Is it every day? Every meal? Maybe it happens more in a particular place or on a particular occasion. It's probably pretty obvious that mind*ful* eaters do exactly the opposite of mind*less* eaters. A good example of mindful eaters are babies. If you give a baby a grape, they don't just eat it straight away, they do literally everything else with it first. They analyse with curiosity how it looks, the shapes, the textures, how it feels, how it smells, they would probably even stick it up their nose before putting it in their mouths. That's basically mindful eating, living totally in the present, noticing everything there is to notice, allowing yourself to be curious, (except you don't have to stick food up your nose).

Keep your attention focused solely on the food and eating. Naturally, our minds love multitasking. They will try to be more 'efficient', and will try to use this time while eating to do other things like, make plans, think of work, remind us of things on the 'to-do' list, worry about literally anything and play that annoying song we can't get out of our heads. This is completely normal so don't get frustrated when this happens, but always try and notice it happening. And when you do notice it, gently bring your attention back to the present sensations you are experiencing with the food. As you read previously, meditation is focusing the mind, and that's exactly what we do when we eat mindfully. We are staying focused on the food we're eating. We pay attention to how the food looks, how it smells, what the texture is like in your hand/in your mouth, what it feels like in your mouth, its flavour. In the beginning you may become distracted more often with the thoughts that appear in your head, but the more you practice mindful eating, the better you will get at it. Eventually it will become natural for you to be more in the present when eating.

Always remember to slow down and take your time when you eat. A lot of us eat so much faster than we realise, especially when we're hungry. It takes about 20 minutes for your brain to register that you're full. So when we eat fast, we're much more likely to eat past the point of fullness. When we eat slowly, we realise our fullness and can stop before we get to the point of overindulging. Slowing down allows you to really be able to notice everything about the food and your experience. It's a more intense experience when we concentrate more, but it often results in us eating less. What's the point in scoffing down a whole bag of Cheetos if you're not even getting 100% of the experience? If you eat them slowly then you enjoy the taste, with less going into your stomach. So, take your time when eating, whenever you can. Avoid eating in front of the tv and sit at a table whenever possible. Sitting at a table automatically encourages you to focus more on the food. Be sure to chew your food thoroughly before swallowing, not only does help you to slow down but digestion starts in the mouth, therefore, the more you chew, the less work your body has to do later on.

Sometimes in daily life we don't always have time to slow down, maybe you have only a five-minute lunch break and don't have the time to eat slowly. In this case I would suggest you at least make a conscious effort to tune in while you eat, chew your food properly and keep your attention present. And be aware, if you're rushing, you may even be eating more than you need. You can get to know how much food your body really needs by paying attention to how much you eat when you do have the time to slow down.

Mindful eating exercise

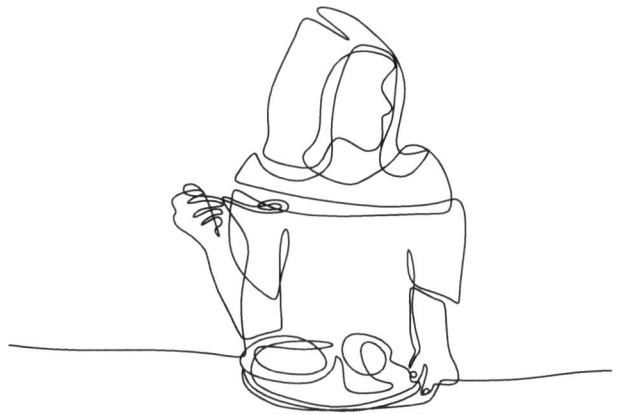

Aim to do the following exercise once a day. It can be with a meal or even with something simple like a grape.

1. Make sure you're in a place you feel comfortable to eat and relaxed with no distractions. For example, at home at the dinner table, phone away and tv off. Sitting upright, spine lengthened (but comfortable) and with your food in front of you.

2. Take a moment first of all to take a mental note of how hungry you are. Rate your hunger and fullness.

3. Inhale the aroma, how does it smell? How does the smell make you feel? Does your mouth salivate? Notice these feelings.

4. How does it look? What do you notice first of all when you look at it? Notice the colours, the different textures.

5. If you're eating with your hands, notice how the food feels. Is it smooth, rough, does it have any bumps on? If you're eating with cutlery, stay present while you cut through the food, is it hard, soft? Easy to cut/stab?

6. As you put the food into your mouth, stay completely present, notice any sensations that arise. How does the food taste? Do you get an urge to eat faster? What flavours appear? What textures do you feel with your tongue?

7. Chew your food thoroughly and slowly throughout the exercise. How soft/crunchy is it to chew?

8. As you continue to eat, your mind will likely wander. When this happens, simply bring it back to focus on the food and continue to notice the flavours, textures and any other sensations as you eat.

9. Avoid judging the food or forming opinions, just notice and accept.

10. Check in with your stomach every so often to feel how full/hungry you are.

Mindful eating tips

1. If you're eating with company or out in a restaurant you won't always be able to concentrate as much as you would in the exercise above. To be more mindful in these situations, while you're eating, every now and again draw your attention to your mouth whilst chewing, and pay attention to the taste and textures. Then check in with sensations your stomach is giving you. How hungry are you? Pause halfway through and take a couple sips of water. Once you begin practicing the mindful eating exercise it will become more of a habit to check in which will help in these situations.

2. Stop for a drink. Always try to keep a glass of water or another drink next to you while you eat. Drinking in between mouthfuls (not every mouthful, but every now and again) naturally slows down your eating, giving your food more time to move through your body, therefore giving your brain more of a chance to realise how full the stomach is.

3. Whenever you can, try and eat with as little distractions as possible. This means avoid being on your phone while eating and avoid watching tv at every meal time. This isn't always possible as sometimes you may not be eating alone, but no matter the situation, be sure to come back to the present moment every so often and mentally check in.

4. Eat with good posture. Eating with good posture is an act of self-love and respect for your body. When we slouch, it affects our whole body, and if it becomes a habit it can even alter our bodies long term e.g. hunchbacks and forward-head posture. Slouching slows down digestion and can encourage acid reflux, as it put pressure on the abdominal. So, be sure that your spine is upright, shoulders are back, and your head and neck are in line with your back (at same time be sure not to strain, you want to be comfortable). Another problem is that many of us unconsciously jolt our necks forward to reach our forks. To encourage good posture, we want to first of all make sure we're sitting close enough to the food, then, when we lean forward to eat, it should come more from the hips then the neck.

5. Notice and embrace any questions or curiosities you have about the food you're eating, where it comes from, how it's made, what is actually in it. You can research the answers to your questions after you've finished eating. It's always useful to educate yourself, especially on something that is affecting something like your body and health so directly.

6. When you have the time, just before you're about to eat, take a moment to clear your mind. Consider where the food that you're about to eat has come from. Maybe you're eating some rice for example, think about all the workers in the rice fields that work long hours out in the mud, growing and harvesting the rice, all the water used to feed the soil, the energy used in the transportation of the rice to your country. Even if you don't know exactly where it comes from, use your imagination (you always research later). So much of our food comes from overseas these days and we're so lucky to be able to eat any food we want at any time of the year, unlike those some generations before us, who were limited to eating only what is in season and available at the time.

7. Say thank you. Before I eat, I like to say a mental prayer, it doesn't matter what religion you are or if you have no religion. You can still thank the universe for providing you with the food that's on your plate and recognise the fact that you have the privilege of eating a meal, unlike so many other people in the world. It doesn't have to take a long time, sometimes I take a couple minutes and really concentrate and sometimes it's more of a 'thank you'. A lot of people when they hear the word prayer think they have to say words, and you can if you want to, but also, feeling, appreciating and acknowledging is a prayer in itself. Below I've created a mindful prayer for you to use as a guide.

Mindful eating prayer

'Thank you, universe, for supplying this earth with such amazing, nutritious and tasty food.

Thank you to all of the workers who contributed in making it possible for me to be able to eat this meal [or name other food here].

Thank you to my body for taking in all of the nutrients, vitamins and goodness that this food has to offer.'

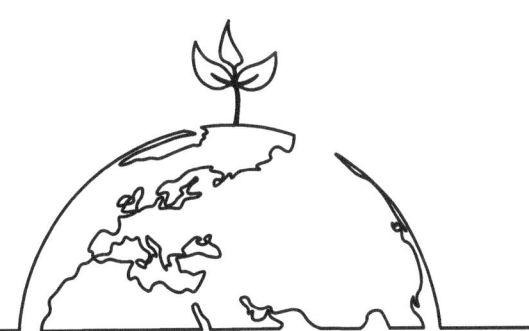

I just want to add whilst we're on the subject of mindful eating and thinking about where our food is coming from that it's worth thinking about where the animal products that you're eating (if you're eating them) are coming from, and the process of how they came to be on your plate. Many people chose to avoid thinking about these things, and I can understand why, when you really think about it, it doesn't exactly put you in the mood to eat it. Why is the process of how a cow came to be on our plate so much less appetising than say, the process of an apple being picked from a tree on an apple farm? It's okay to ask why, you might ask why and conclude that you are still happy to continue eating meat. That's fine. I'm not here trying to change your opinion, I'm just trying to (hopefully) help you to make the decision consciously. Because if we keep our eyes closed to something, and just continue doing it out of habit, then we're not actually making that decision ourselves, we're living in a way which someone else has taught us to (our parents, our culture etc.). We're acting through their beliefs not our own.

I was raised in a big Italian family in the UK and growing up eating countless beef lasagnes, salami sandwiches and meatballs, I was never taught to think twice about where the meat I ate come. I never really saw it as an actual animal, or something that was once a living, breathing thing. I was completely unaware. I had no idea which meat was even in the meatballs I ate, or that pork was coming from a pig and not a cow. Clueless. Then around the age of 22 I began to question where exactly it came from and the process the animal goes through. I did some research and opened my eyes up to a whole world of (unpleasant) things that were just so casually swept under the rug. Such as the conditions that the animals are kept in, the processed food and chemicals they're fed, and how they are treated and killed. I genuinely couldn't believe I had gone 22 years of my life just mindlessly consuming all this meat without ever thinking twice about it, and my whole entire family the same. There's so much more out there to learn on the subject (I'm just touching on it lightly). But I knew from that moment I had to educate myself about it more to really be able to make the right decision. I wanted to live the rest of my life knowing that what I eat doesn't cause unnecessary harm to others, or the planet which my future children and grandchildren will greatly rely on, and just as importantly, I wanted to live a long, healthy life.

I considered the fact that although our bodies are anatomically herbivorous, humans clearly evolved to eat meat. However it's safe to say that, when our ancestors were hunting animals, it was somewhat a 'fair fight,' there was a 50:50 chance for the animal to escape and survive, and also a fair chance that us humans would be hunted by other predators. We were a part of the animal kingdom. Now, although we are technically still part of it, we have totally separated ourselves from it. We select the ones that we deem as cute or acceptable to live amongst us, and we choose not to associate ourselves generally with any animal that we consider food. We then contain and breed these animals we've labelled as food for this sole purpose, and every aspect of their lives are controlled from start to finish. Still sound like a fair fight?

Through my own research and contemplation, I have come to a settlement which I believe I can live happily and healthily. I didn't change overnight, believe me. It took a couple of years (and a lot of regretted drunk McDonald's cheeseburgers) to fully get here. But I now no longer eat meat, I mostly avoid cheese and dairy (I would like to say totally but that would be untrue), I cook plant-based at home and I eat a little fish on the occasion. I also try to make sure most things I eat are organic. That's how I have decided to live my life, I feel good about it, I'm comfortable with it, and I feel healthier than ever. I'm not saying it's the *right* way to live, and I'm not telling you that you should do the same, but what you should do, is take the time to think about it, and make the decision of what you feel is right yourself. All of the recipes included in this book are plant-based, not just for the animals, but also for the health of our own beings. You don't have to be a hardcore vegan to benefit from incorporating a few more fruits and vegetables into your diet, or substituting some processed foods for more whole, natural ones.

TAKE AWAY

Mindful eating plays a key role in Intuitive Eating as it helps us stay in tune with our bodies, trains our minds to be in the present moment and helps us reconnect with the planet.

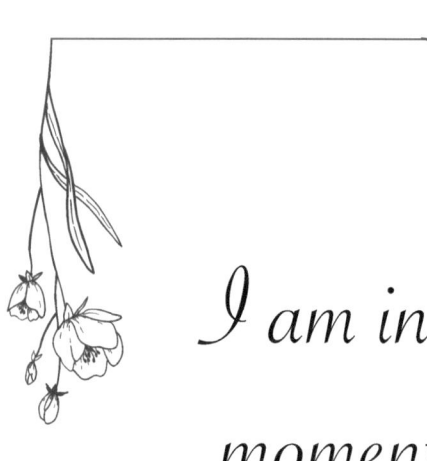

I am in tune with the present moment and grateful for the food I eat

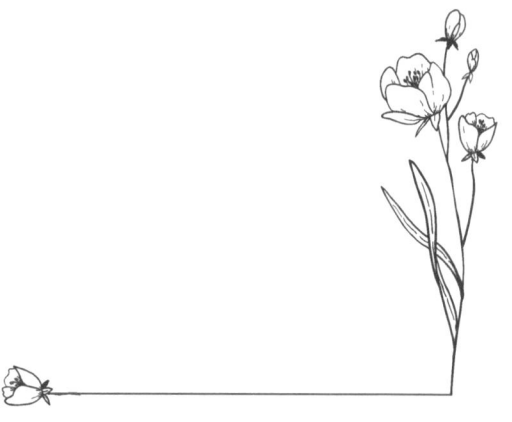

Self-love and self-acceptance

You may think this could be asking too much of you to accept yourself. *All* of yourself. To accept doesn't necessarily mean to *like* every part of yourself, but by accepting something, you are making peace with it and appreciating it simply for what it is and not what you want it to be. The reason this is so important is because this *is* you. Whether you like it or not, this is how you are right now, in this moment in time. Why waste good energy being frustrated about something that you simply cannot change? Not right now anyway. Say you really want to change your hairstyle, but your hairdresser can't fit you in for another two weeks. What do you do? Do you get really mad about it, feel ashamed, hide away until your appointment? Most likely not. You'd probably accept that you have to wait a while before you get your haircut and until then, this will be your hairstyle. This is no different, you are not able to change yourself straight away, the very moment you decide you don't like something. So instead of getting worked up over it, treat it like a haircut. 'It looks like this now and in the future, it may look completely different.' You may, for example, feel insecure about your arms. So instead of looking in the mirror and thinking 'I hate my arms so much, I wish they were thinner,' think (or say aloud) 'I accept that these are my arms today.'

I'm all for affirmations, and I believe when used correctly they can be a very powerful tool, but the truth is, affirmations only work if you *believe* them. Sometimes, when you've felt a certain way about something for a long period of time it's not so easy to convince yourself the opposite. If you keep trying to tell yourself something that you don't believe, a certain frustration can build up, which then actually works in contrast to the effect you are trying to achieve. Looking in the mirror and repeating 'I love arms, I love my arms, I love my a...' after years of trying to hide or change them, can be difficult to even say, let alone believe. But if you begin by looking at them in a different, more realistic, light – e.g. 'My arms are healthy', 'My arms are useful and strong', 'I use them all day long and they allow me to do my job', 'I'm lucky to have two working arms'. If you feel your stomach is not how you want it to look try saying, 'My stomach is such an important organ in my body', 'My stomach works hard to digest my food every day.' Because this *is* the truth, you're not lying to yourself, trying to convince yourself that you feel something you don't, but at the same time, you're also showing appreciation for what you currently have. Sometimes we forget these things because we're so fixated on what we want and what we aren't instead.

It's important to remind ourselves of these things because the fact of the matter is, we are lucky for what we have now, and if we can't appreciate what we have, how can we possibly begin to ask for more? If you're someone who believes in manifestation then you will know already that it's the emotion behind what you're asking for that really matters. So if you're using affirmations with a background of built up anger, frustration and other low vibrational feelings, then you may as well try manifesting the sky to turn green and the clouds to turn purple – it's not gonna happen. By accepting ourselves as we are we take away the anger and frustration and we, at the very least, become neutral towards these areas which we feel most insecure about – we remove the negative feelings. There is no inner peace when you don't accept yourself. How can there be, when it's you *against* your body? The fight will only end once you accept yourself. You will feel lighter and you can finally relax. Instead of seeing things through a judgmental perspective, worried about how you feel it 'should' look, you're seeing it for what it actually is. Nothing more, nothing less.

When you begin to accept myself, you will notice that the little things don't bother you so much anymore. When you don't accept yourself, you feel the need to try and change immediately, skipping the next meal, starving yourself, killing yourself in the gym that day, looking for shortcuts. The problem with this is, it's simply not sustainable. Just because you skip a meal won't make you any skinnier,

skip a few meals and yes you may lose a little weight, although it won't necessarily be good for you. But anyway, how long can it last? In my experience, when you charge headfirst into something in a 'extreme' way, it never lasts. And cosmetic procedures can only get you so far, if you've had one already, you'll know that *literally* nothing can replace a healthy lifestyle. But by accepting yourself as you are now, you stop the irrational craving of wanting to change overnight and you put yourself in the right mindset to achieve long-term goals.

Just because you're accepting your current situation does not mean you're giving up or giving in and it definitely doesn't mean you can't try to change it. It will actually help you get to where you want to be even faster. It's fine to want to change or improve something. Change is an inevitable part of life and your body will change weather you like it or not. So why not decide how it changes, you do have a large say in this. For example, yes people age, but how are you going to age? There are many people out there who are in better shape in their 40s than they were in their earlier years. Because even at a later age, they decided to eat more nourishing foods and workout more. They're classic examples of people who decided how their bodies will change. Pregnant women who make the effort to eat well and stay active during pregnancy and after childbirth are choosing how their bodies will change. Young people who move out from their childhood homes and learn to cook for themselves are also choosing how they will change. There's nothing wrong with wanting to change things, lose or gain a little weight and become a healthier person. Just make sure you're doing this for *you*. Don't spend time worrying about images in magazines and on social media, or what is currently considered the latest trend (e.g. small boobs, skinny, big boobs, big bum, full bodied), because these things are always going to change. Do what *you* want to do. Eat what *you* want to eat and look how *you* want to look. When our intention is to seek the approval of others, we can never truly be happy, because, once their opinions change (which they always will) and fashion trends change, we find we no longer fit into what is acceptable, and once again we find ourselves back where we started, chasing approval. To truly be happy we must start with ourselves, do things for ourselves, achieve things for ourselves, love ourselves and accept ourselves as we are.

Once you've made peace with your body you can begin to set realistic goals. These goals will be different to before as there will be no pressure attached to them. No time limit or dead line to achieve them by. You accept and appreciate your body as it is now, so there's no rush. Make sure your health is a priority when you set your goals. Maybe you're content with how you are and your goal is to maintain your current body in a healthy way or maybe you want to be more toned. It's not only about how you look but also how you feel, perhaps you want more stamina and you want more energy. Whatever it is, don't hesitate to take

steps in that direction, but do it with the health of your being as the main focus point. By eating intuitively you'll find your body will change naturally into a more healthful state. For some that will mean losing weight and for others that will mean gaining some weight, but so long as we are listening to our bodies and choosing to eat nourishing foods, we can always be sure that the change will be a positive one.

Why are we so hard on ourselves anyway? Does it boil down to the fact that we think other people won't like what they see? If it were just you, all alone on this planet, would you really care about the fact your waistline is a bit larger than what you felt was socially acceptable, that your hair needs brushing or your legs need shaving or that your wearing odd socks today. I know I wouldn't. In fact, I'd probably enjoy it. Imagine that, a world where you didn't have to give a flying f*ck about what you look like or what other people think. I'm not saying you shouldn't brush your hair or you have to walk around with hairy legs and odd socks on, but what I'm saying is that, fundamentally, do you even *really* care about these things? What would you spend your energy on if you weren't using up so much of it worrying about what other people see? By worrying about what other people think, you are placing your happiness in their hands. When someone approves of you, you feel good, when someone's disapproves, you feel bad. Their opinion of you is deciding how you feel. You give them a power over that you that no one should have, except you. Whenever you're in a situation and an insecure thought comes into your head, remind yourself of this. They can't decide how you feel, only you can truly decide this. Sure, other people will have their opinions, but it's how you process and retaliate to their opinions that will ultimately affect you, not their opinion itself. An opinion without a reaction becomes completely meaningless. And anyway, do you really want to be loved for your flat stomach, or do you want to be loved for who you are as a person and how you make other people around you feel when they're around you?

The reason why I speak about self-love in an Intuitive Eating recipe book, is because, Intuitive Eating isn't just about food, it's about your whole lifestyle. That includes your mentality, the clothes you wear, the places you go to, the people you choose to hang out with and even the conversations that you have. To really be at peace and in tune with yourself, everything else in your life should also align with this. This will happen somewhat naturally as you practise your meditations and mindfulness exercises, but you may also find yourself making changes to your current life and deciding to do things differently to before. For example, you might find yourself wearing different clothes to before because you now chose to wear clothes that fit you in a more comfortable way, rather than clothes that 'suck you in' in certain places. You might find you're more aware of negative talk, and prefer to avoid conversations which criticise the way other people look, this may also affect the people who you chose to surround yourself with. You may choose to eat in different restaurants and therefore hang out in different places to before. Your goals in life may well change completely, and you'll have so much more energy from the meditation to achieve them. Your mind will be a more peaceful and loving place and with this new mentality other aspects of your life will inevitably change.

TAKEAWAY

Intuitive Eating is also about accepting and appreciating your body as well as being open to changes in life which align with your new mindset.

I cherish my body as it is today
and I appreciate all it does for me

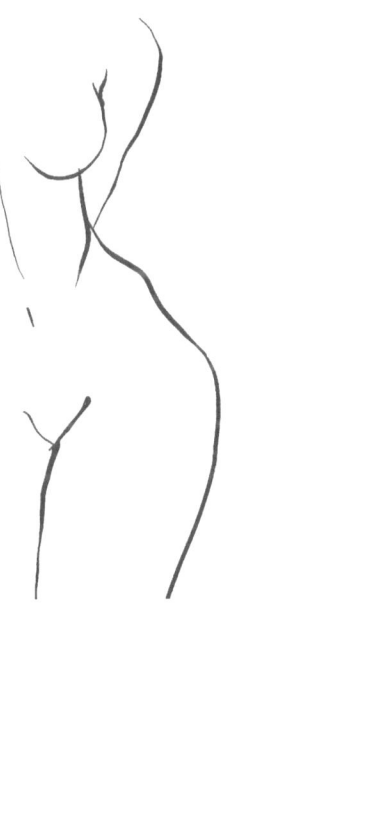

Mind-to-body meditation

This mediation is great for getting back in touch with your body. I like to do this whenever I have a spare few minutes in my day, I often do it when I'm travelling in the car (passenger seat) or on a plane. You can do it for just a few minutes or you can spend longer doing it, 10–15 minutes. Just make sure you're sat or laid down in a comfortable position and follow the steps below.

1. Begin by closing your eyes, focusing your awareness on your toes and working your way up your feet. Notice how they feel, are they touching something? Any time a thought comes into your head, gently shift your focus back to your feet.

2. Slowly bring your attention up to your legs, also noticing what you feel, are your clothes touching them anywhere? Are they touching the chair or bed? Any time you feel your mind begin to wonder, gently bring it back to the body part you were focusing on.

3. Continue scanning your attention upwards, from your calves to your thighs, up to your hips, stomach, chest, do you feel you heart beating? Focus on your shoulders, on to your arms (each arm individually if you have time), your neck and then head.

4. Continue throughout the practice, shifting your mind back to the body every time it begins to wonder. If you come across a body part and notice it's tense then simply relax it, and then move on.

Spread the message

One of the most important parts of being an Intuitive Eater, is to spread the message and share the knowledge. This doesn't mean you have to go around announcing it to people or bore everyone with long speeches, but there are so many situations in daily life, where we have the power to encourage or discourage diet culture promoting behaviours. There are things that most of us have been guilty of doing in the past that contribute to the encouragement of the diet culture without even realising. We've all told that friend that they look so skinny after they've told us how they've been restricting themselves so much on their new diet (we congratulate them even). Some of us have made comments on another person's weight, mocked or laughed at jokes made about people with a different body shape to ours, we might be promoting diet products online by posting about them on social media, even just by participating in conversations about diets/weight loss can be promoting diet culture behaviour. One option is to stay silent when some of these situations arise, this way at least you are not contributing. The second option is to share a new point of view, communicate and inform people of Intuitive Eating, in a calm and positive manner. People think and act the way that they do because that's more than likely the only way they have learned to behave, so why not teach them something new? This can be by simply using yourself as an example, sharing your experience. Telling them how eating intuitively has worked for you. Let them know that when you eat intuitively, you learn to love yourself and be proud of who you are. You free yourself of the stress and pressure to look a certain way, you let go of the fear of judgment, nor do you feel the need to judge others, and that by listening to your body, you are able to maintain a healthy, fulfilling lifestyle, which not only allows you to actually enjoy food, but benefits your health, and that you look, and feel amazing because of it.

TAKEAWAY

Spread the message, share the love.

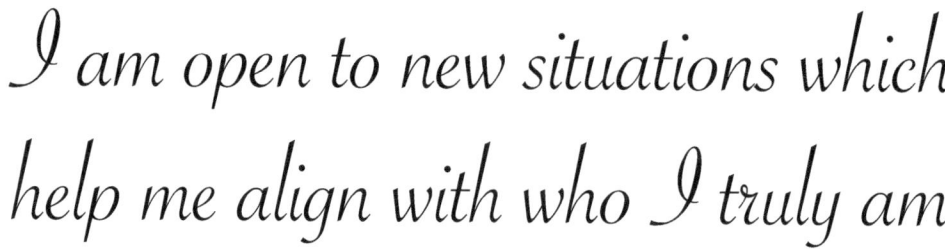

I am open to new situations which help me align with who I truly am

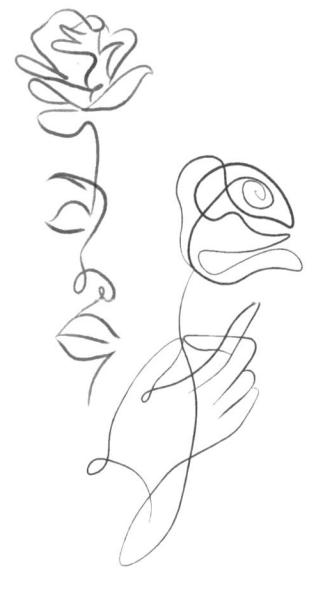

RECIPES

The recipes in this book are made from natural, whole, plant-based foods which include as many fruits and veggies as possible.

We will be using these healthful ingredients to recreate some of our typical favorite foods whilst maintaining their great taste, and also to create delicious breakfast, lunches and dinners.

Convenience and simplicity are the key to making these recipes become part of our daily lives. By using such simple ingredients and straightforward cooking techniques we can incorporate these dishes easily with our daily routines.

By eating this type of food, we can be sure that we are doing the best thing for the health of our own bodies, other animals, and the planet.

Bon' apetit

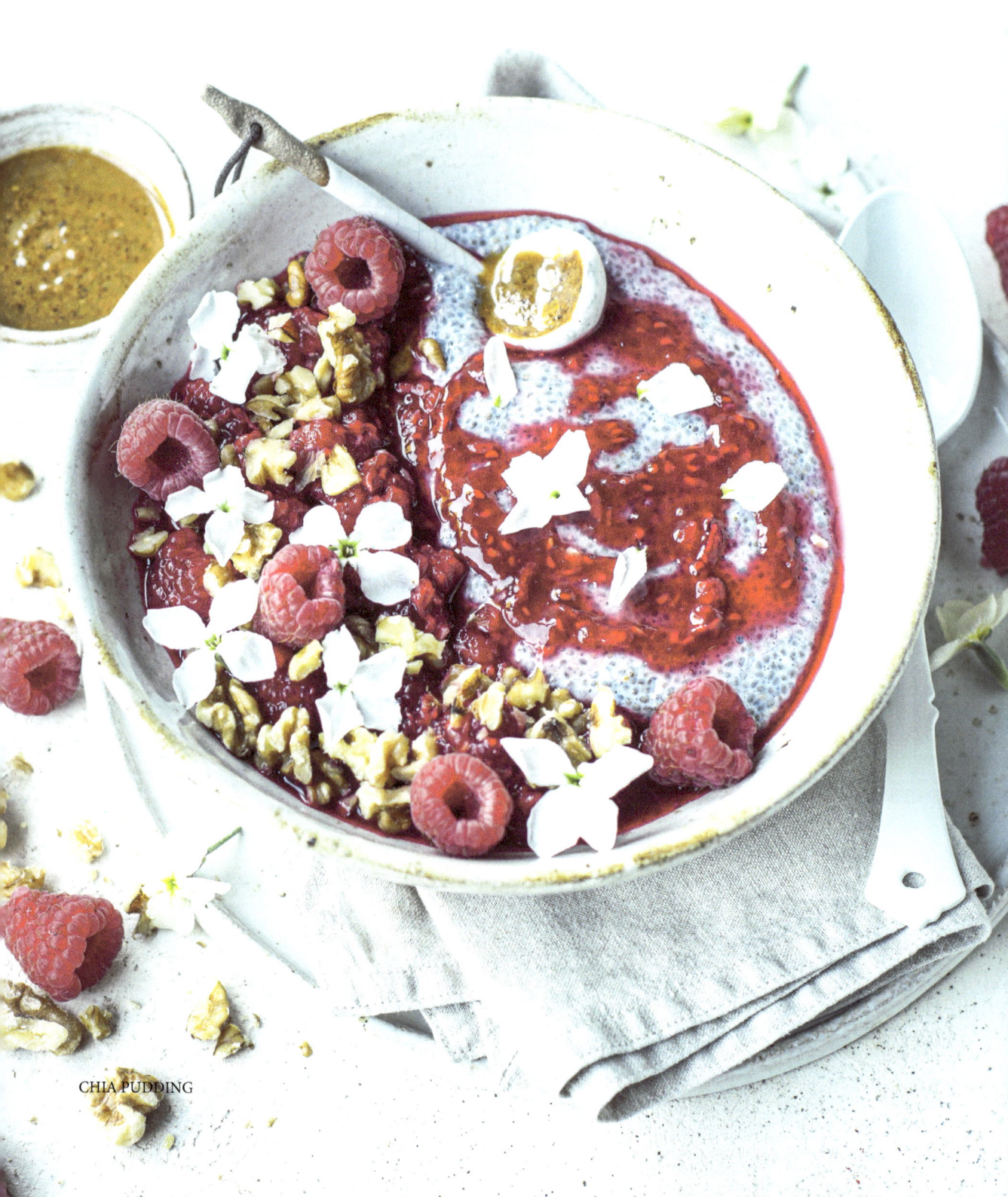

CHIA PUDDING

CHIA PUDDING

I love how simple this recipe is and yet so tasty. It's great to eat in the morning because the high fibre content from the chia seeds and raspberries leads to slower digestion and lasting satiety. The combination of the zing from the raspberries and ginger goes beautifully with the mild flavour and creamy texture of the coconut chia pudding.

Ingredients
200ml coconut milk
3 tbsp chia seeds
Sprinkle salt
100g raspberry
2cm grated ginger

Topping:
Small handful crushed walnuts
1 tbsp almond butter

STEP 1
Shake coconut milk well before opening, then pour it into a bowl. Mix in the chia seeds and salt. Stir well and leave to one side.

STEP 2
Add the raspberries and mash slightly some of them with a fork. Add the ginger and stir. Turn on medium heat and let the raspberries heat up for 2–5 minutes, do not boil them.

STEP 3
Pour the raspberry mixture onto the chia pudding and add toppings as desired.

DID YOU KNOW:
Chia seeds are a great source of ALA Omega 3. Omega 3 helps with heart function, brain function, inflammatory responses and lowering blood sugar. There are three main types of omega 3, ALA (mostly found in plants), EPA and DHA (mostly found in oily fish), however, our bodies are actually capable of converting a small amount of ALA omega 3 into the other two.

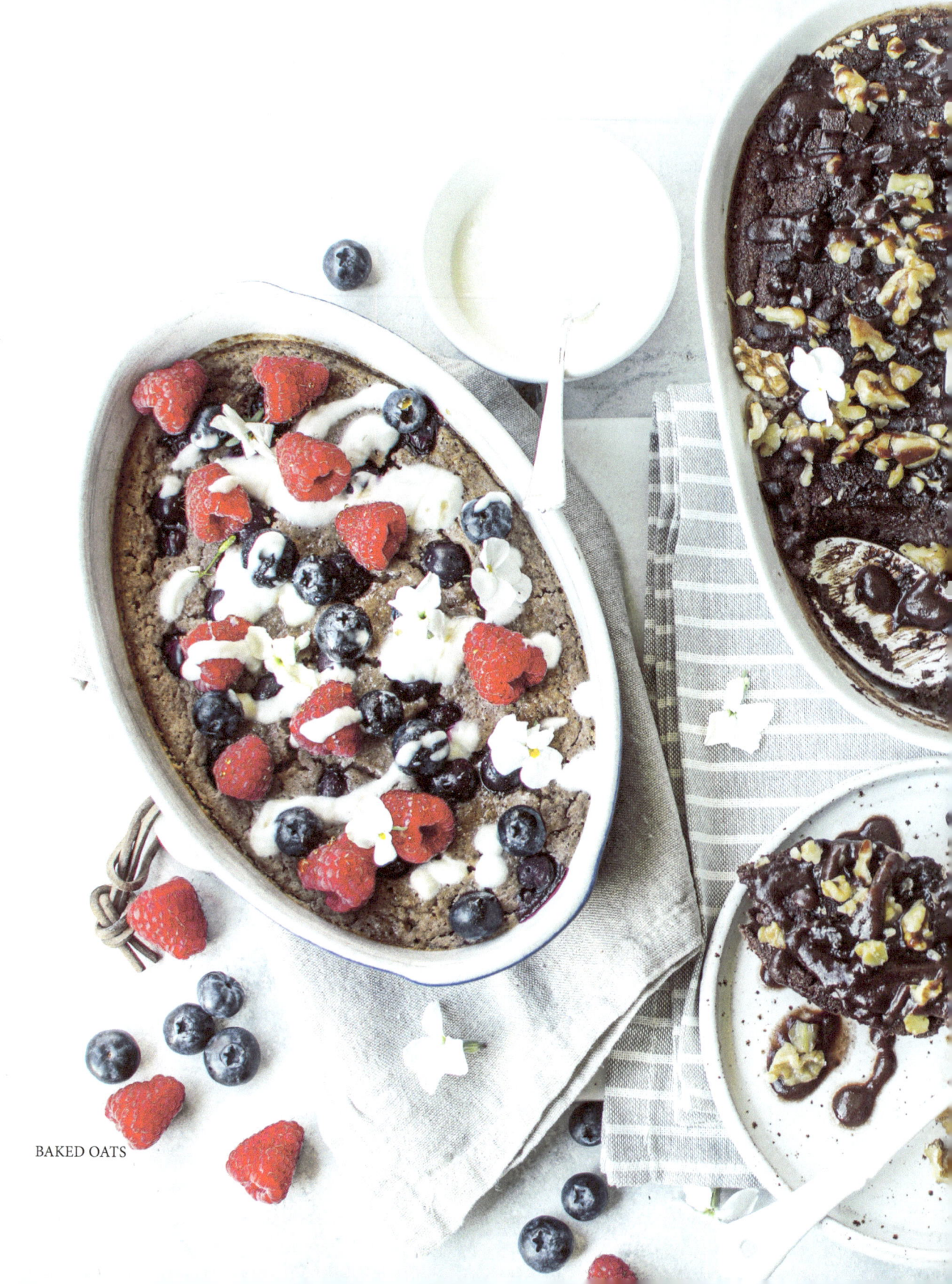

BAKED OATS

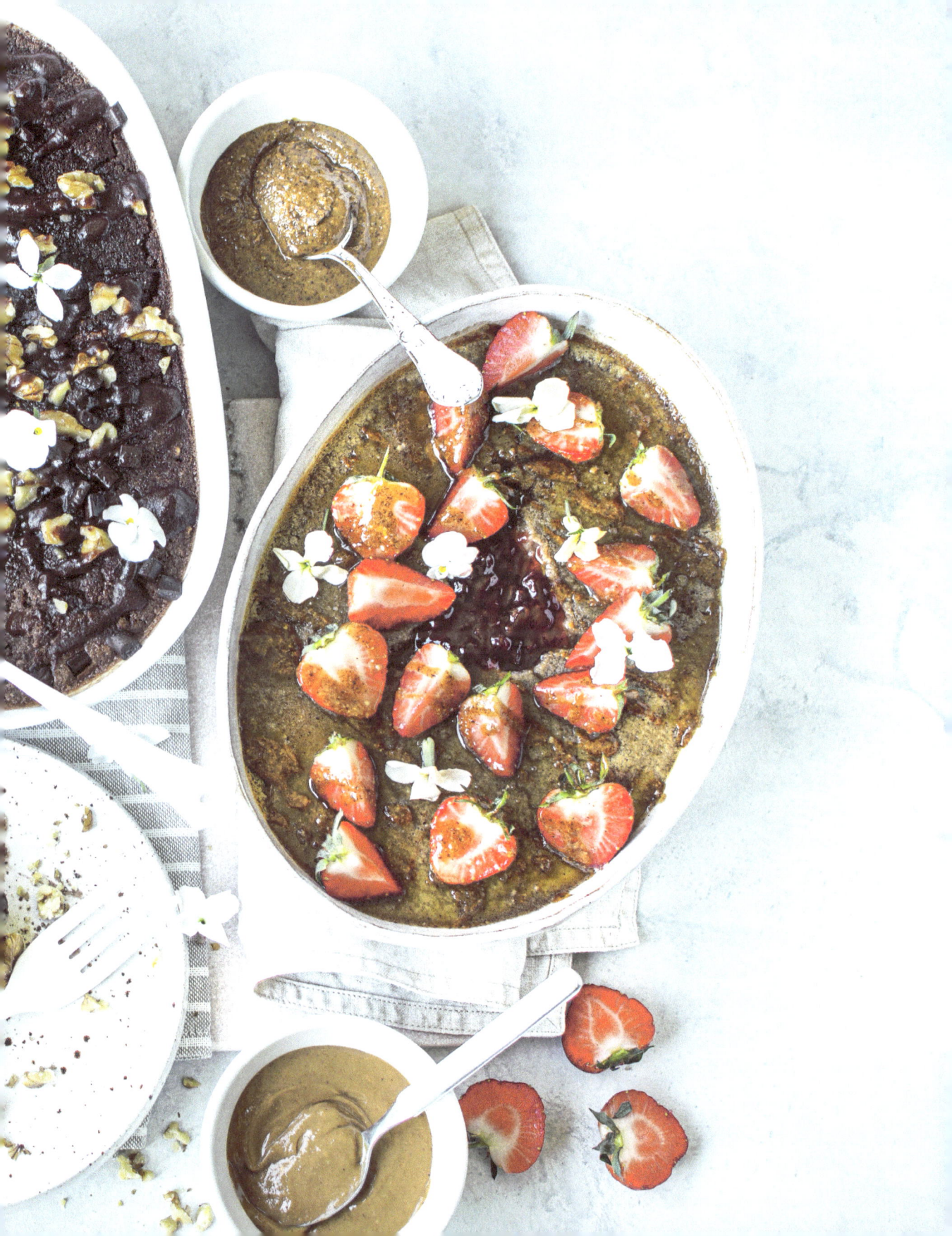

BAKED OATS

SERVES 1 PERSON

Oat are a highly nutritious way to start your day, packed with vitamins, minerals and antioxidants. They're also high in fibre and contain more protein than other grains, giving you a lasting fullness and slow burning energy. Plus, these baked oats are absolutely delicious.

Chocolate delight

1 cup oats
2 tsp cocoa powder
1 tbsp hazelnut butter
½ tsp baking powder
1 tbsp maple syrup
1 tsp chia seeds
1¼ cup oat milk
Small handful of dark choc chips

Creamy chocolate sauce

2–3 dates
10 tbsp boiling water
1 tbsp coconut cream
1 tsp coco powder
Sprinkle salt

Toppings (optional)

nuts
chocolate chips

STEP 1
Preheat oven to 180 degrees. Combine all of the baked oats ingredients together in a blender except the chocolate chips, and blend. Then stir in the chocolate chips.

STEP 2
Pour into baking tin and put in the oven for 25–30 minutes.

STEP 3
Whilst the oats are baking, combine all of the sauce ingredient in the blender and blend until smooth.

STEP 4
Remove oats from oven. Pour on sauce and add toppings.

Summer berry with coconut and ginger yogurt

1 cup oats
1¼ cup almond milk
1 tbsp almond butter
½ tsp baking powder
1 tbsp maple syrup
1 tsp chia seeds
1 vanilla pod
40g raspberries
40g blueberries

Ginger & coconut yogurt

1–2 tbsp coconut yogurt
2cm inch grated ginger

Toppings

Blueberries and raspberries
Top with cashew or almond butter

STEP 1
Preheat oven to 180 degrees. Combine all of the baked oats mixture together except the blueberries and blend. Then stir in the blueberries.

STEP 2
Pour into baking tin and put in the oven for 25–30 minutes.

STEP 3
Whilst the oats are baking, combine the coconut yogurt and ginger together in a bowl and stir well.

STEP 4
Remove oats from oven. Top with yogurt, berries and nut butter.

Jam doughnut

1 cup oats
1 ¼ cup oat milk
1 tsp chia seeds
1 vanilla
1 tbsp cashew butter
1 tbsp maple syrup
½ tsp baking powder
1 tsp heaped Strawberry jam

Toppings

Cashew butter
Handful of chopped fresh strawberries

STEP 1
Preheat oven to 180 degrees. Combine all of the baked oats mixture together except the strawberry jam and blend. Then pour into baking tin.

STEP 2
Add the heaped spoon of jam directly into the middle of the mixture in the baking tin.

STEP 3
Place baking tin in the oven and bake for 25–30 minutes.

STEP 4
Remove oats from oven. Top with berries and nut butter.

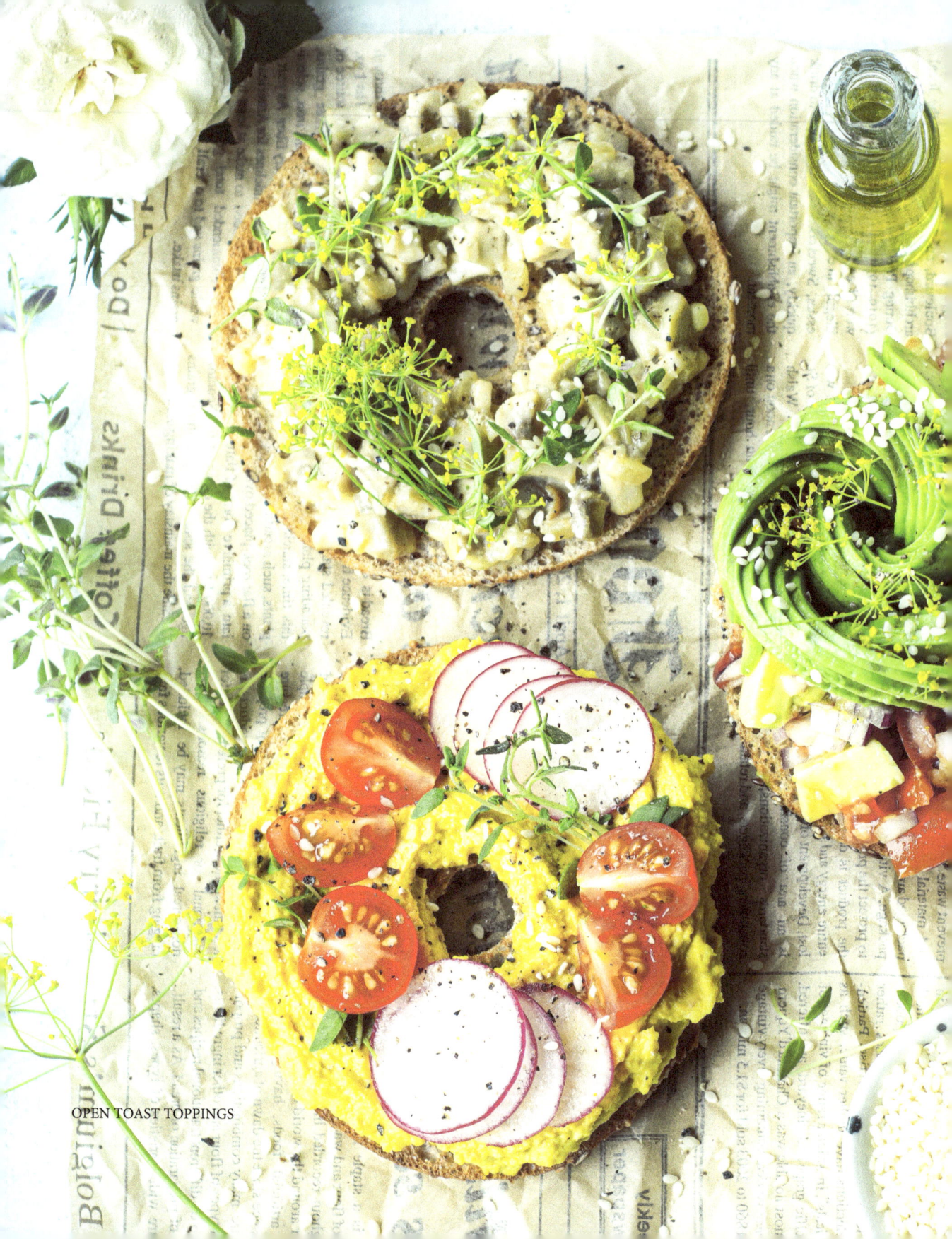

OPEN TOAST TOPPINGS

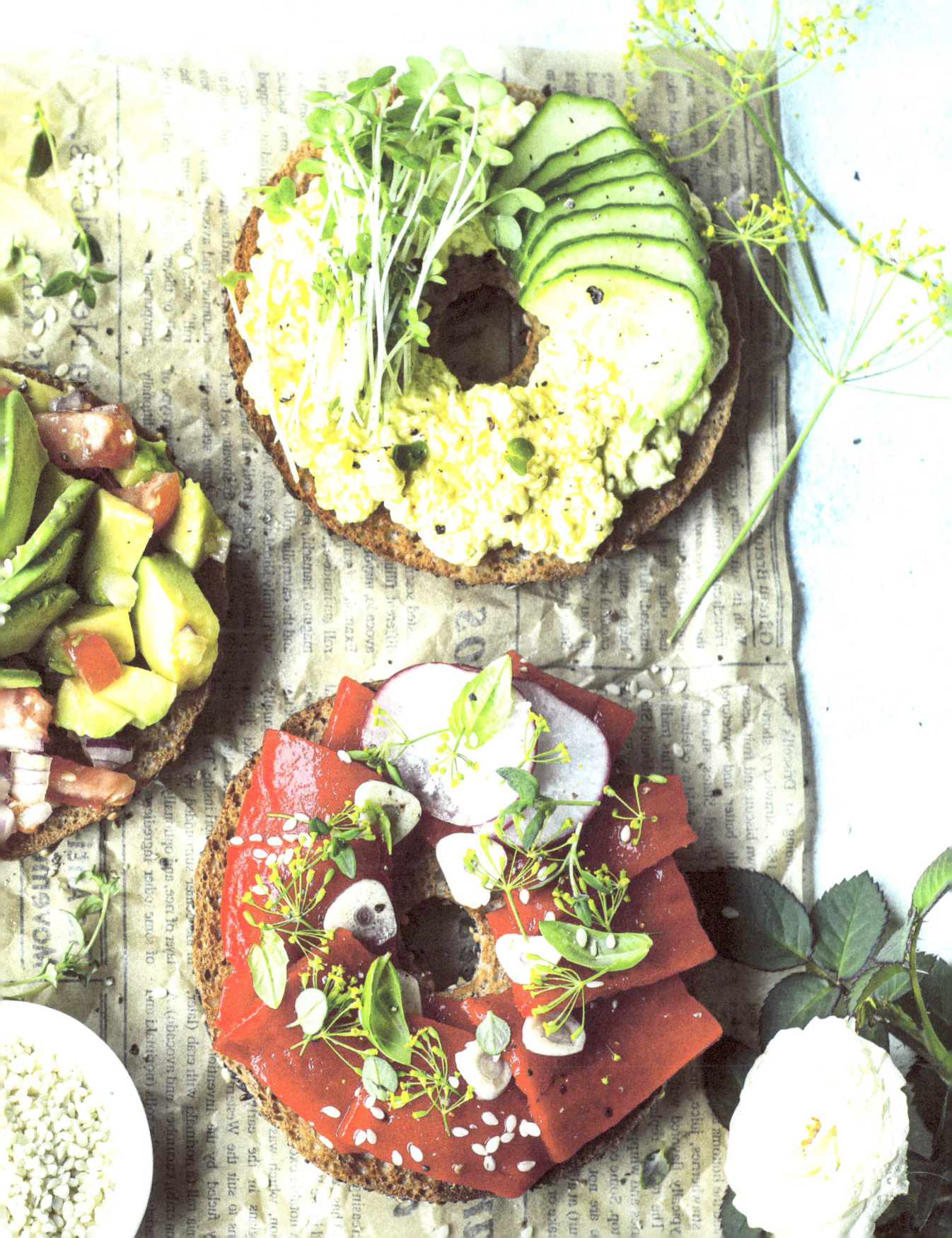

OPEN TOAST TOPPINGS

I love a toast topping, perfect for any time of the day when you're feeling peckish. These toppings are all super simple to make and can be stored in an airtight container in the fridge for a couple of days.

Avocado, tomato + ginger one

1 avocado
½ red onion
1 tomato
2cm grated ginger
1 tbsp olive
Salt

STEP 1
Chop avocado into small bite size pieces and chop red onion.

STEP 2
Add all the ingredients into a bowl and stir together well.

Creamy Mushroom one

Half an onion
1 garlic clove
100g button mushrooms (can use any other)
4–5 tbsp coconut milk from carton
1 tsp nutritional yeast
Top with chives or parsley

STEP 1
Chop up garlic and onion and fry in a pan with some oil for about 2–3 minutes. Then chop up and add mushrooms.

STEP 2
Once mushrooms are cooked turn heat to low. Add the coconut milk, nutritional yeast and salt. Stir well and add herbs.

Scrambled cheesy tofu

200g silken tofu – patted dry to remove excess water.
¼ tsp onion powder (adjust to taste)
1 heaped tbsp nutritional yeast
Pinch turmeric for colour
Salt

STEP 1
Heat some oil in a frying pan on a medium heat. Add tofu, onion powder, nutritional yeast, turmeric and salt to the pan and stir well (breaking up the tofu).

STEP 2
Cook for about 5 minutes or until any excess water from the tofu has evaporated.

Roast peppers

3–4 bell peppers
Olive oil
1 garlic raw
Salt

STEP 1
Pre-heat oven to 180 degrees. Place peppers on a baking tray in the oven and cook for about 40 minutes (until the skin is slightly burnt and begun to separate from the rest of the pepper).

STEP 2
Remove peppers from oven and let cool for about 15 minutes.

STEP 3
Peel the skin off peppers and put the flesh of the peppers into a separate bowl. Discard of the skin, stalks and seeds.

STEP 4
Chop garlic and add to the bowl of peppers, then cover peppers in olive oil. Add salt, stir and serve.

Turmeric hummus

500g chickpeas
1 garlic clove
5 tbsp olive oil
½ tsp turmeric
Salt
Pepper

STEP 1
Add all ingredients into a blender and blend until smooth.

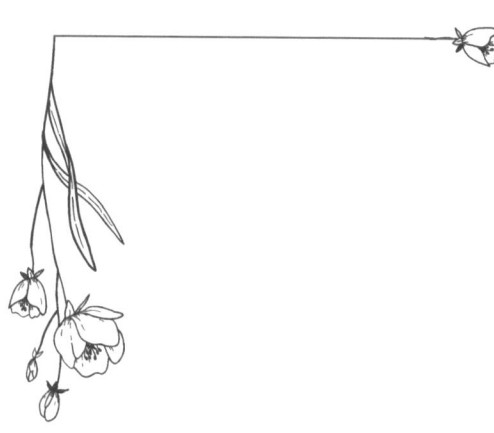

Food is a gift and I allow
myself to enjoy it

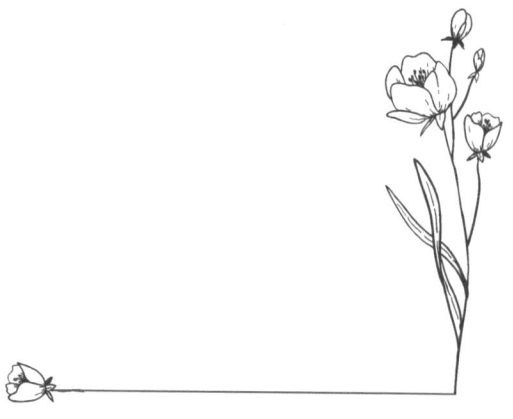

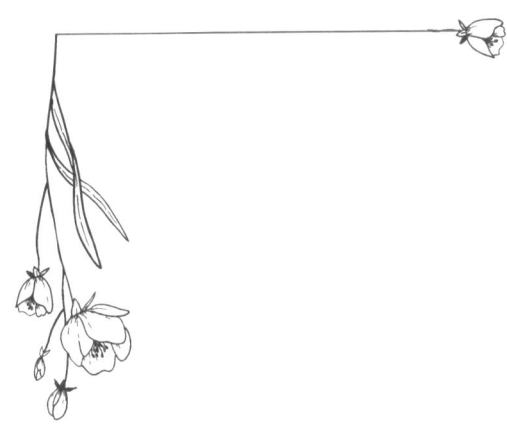

My intention is to maintain good
health and live a long, happy life

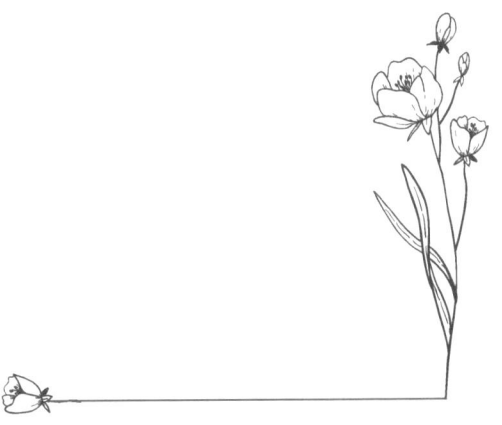

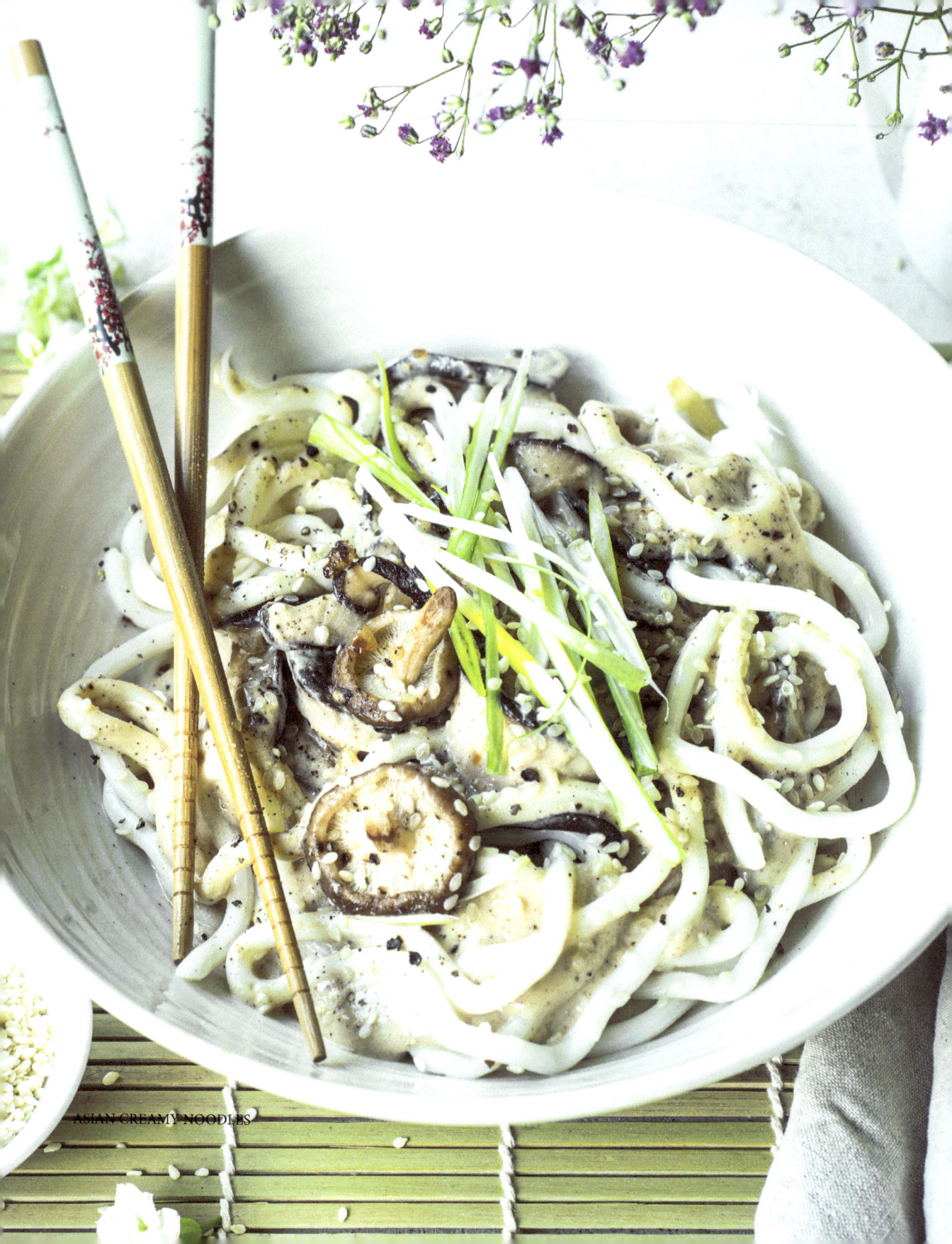

ASIAN CREAMY NOODLES

ASIAN CREAMY NOODLES

SERVES 2–3 PEOPLE

This is a lovely comfort food as it's so creamy and fulfilling. It's also a nice easy recipe for when you're not in the mood to cook a huge meal but want something tasty.

Ingredients

Noodles
200g udon noodles
1 onion
2 garlic cloves
40g dried shiitake mushrooms (soaked)

Sauce
400g coconut yoghurt
1 heaped tbsp almond butter
1 teaspoon brown rice miso paste
2 tbsp nutritional yeast
2 teaspoons tamari
2 teaspoon rice vinegar
Salt and pepper

STEP 1
Boil water in a saucepan and add noodles.

STEP 2
Chop up onion and garlic and fry in a pan on medium heat for 2–3 minutes. Then add mushrooms and cook for further 5 minutes until mushrooms are cooked.

STEP 3
Add all of the sauce ingredients into a blender and blend until thoroughly mixed.

STEP 4
Drain noodles once cooked and add them into the frying pan. Pour sauce on top. Stir together well, and serve.

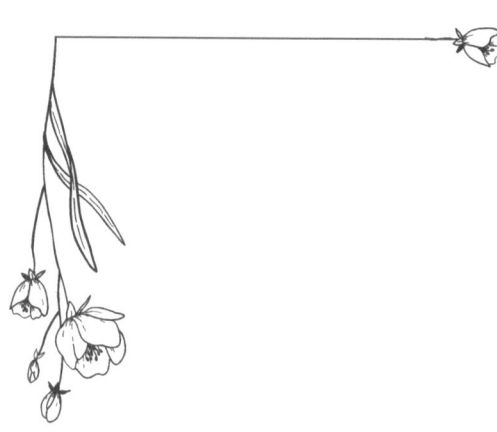

My mind is a calm and
peaceful place

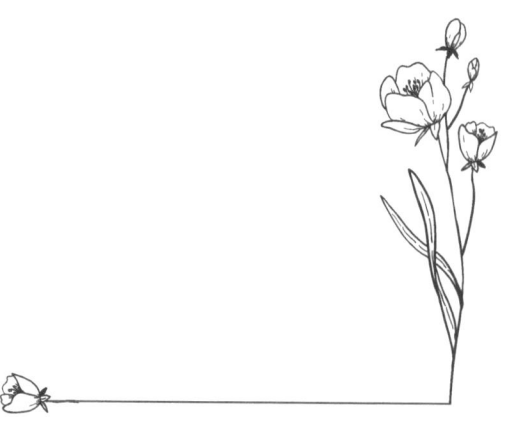

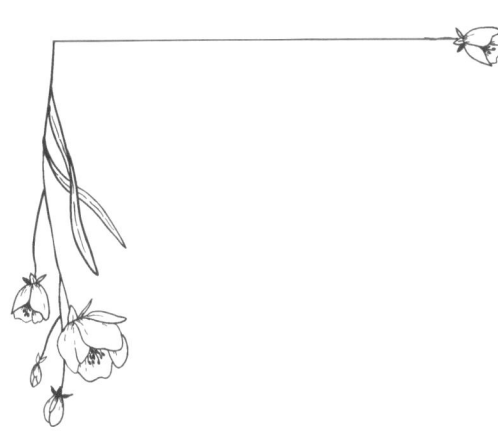

I love and accept myself
as I am today

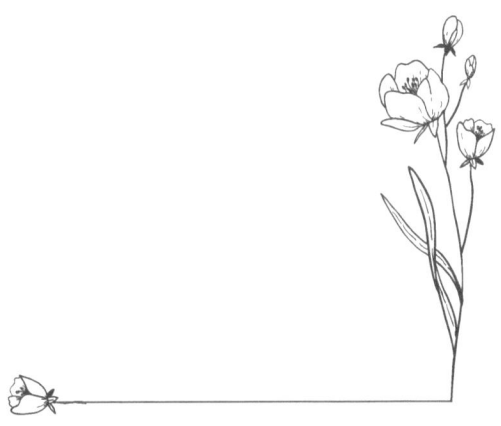

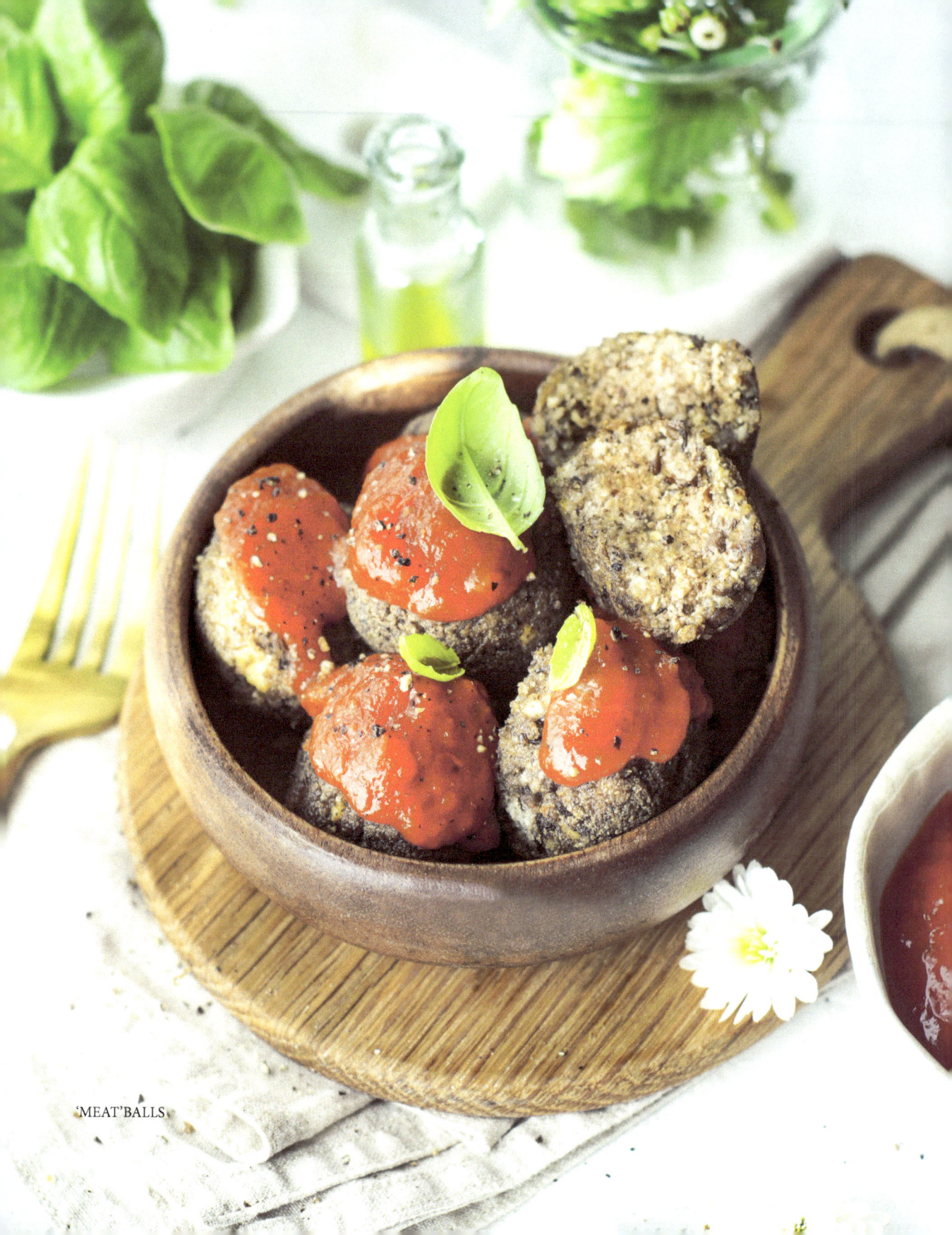

'MEAT'BALLS

'MEAT' BALLS

MAKES 8-12

With all the fake meat on the market these days it's probably not so tempting to make your own, however it's a great feeling knowing all the ingredients are so healthful and nutritious when you make it yourself. Pulses, quinoa and tofu are all excellent forms of protein which makes this recipe great for anyone following a plant-based diet.

1 cup cooked black lentils

½ cup quinoa
170g firm tofu pressed
1 tbsp olive oil
1 tsp garlic powder
1 tsp onion powder
Salt
Pepper

STEP 1
Preheat oven to 180 degrees. Place all ingredients in a blender and blend until thoroughly mixed but still a bit grainy.

STEP 2
Take a small handful of the mixture, roll into a ball and place onto baking tray. Repeat this until all the mixture is used up.

STEP 3
Place baking tray in the oven and cook for 20–30 minutes, until lightly toasting on top.

———————————— TIP ————————————

Serve with the classic tomato sauce (see page 126) and spaghetti of your choice. I often use a black bean spaghetti as an alternative to actual pasta.

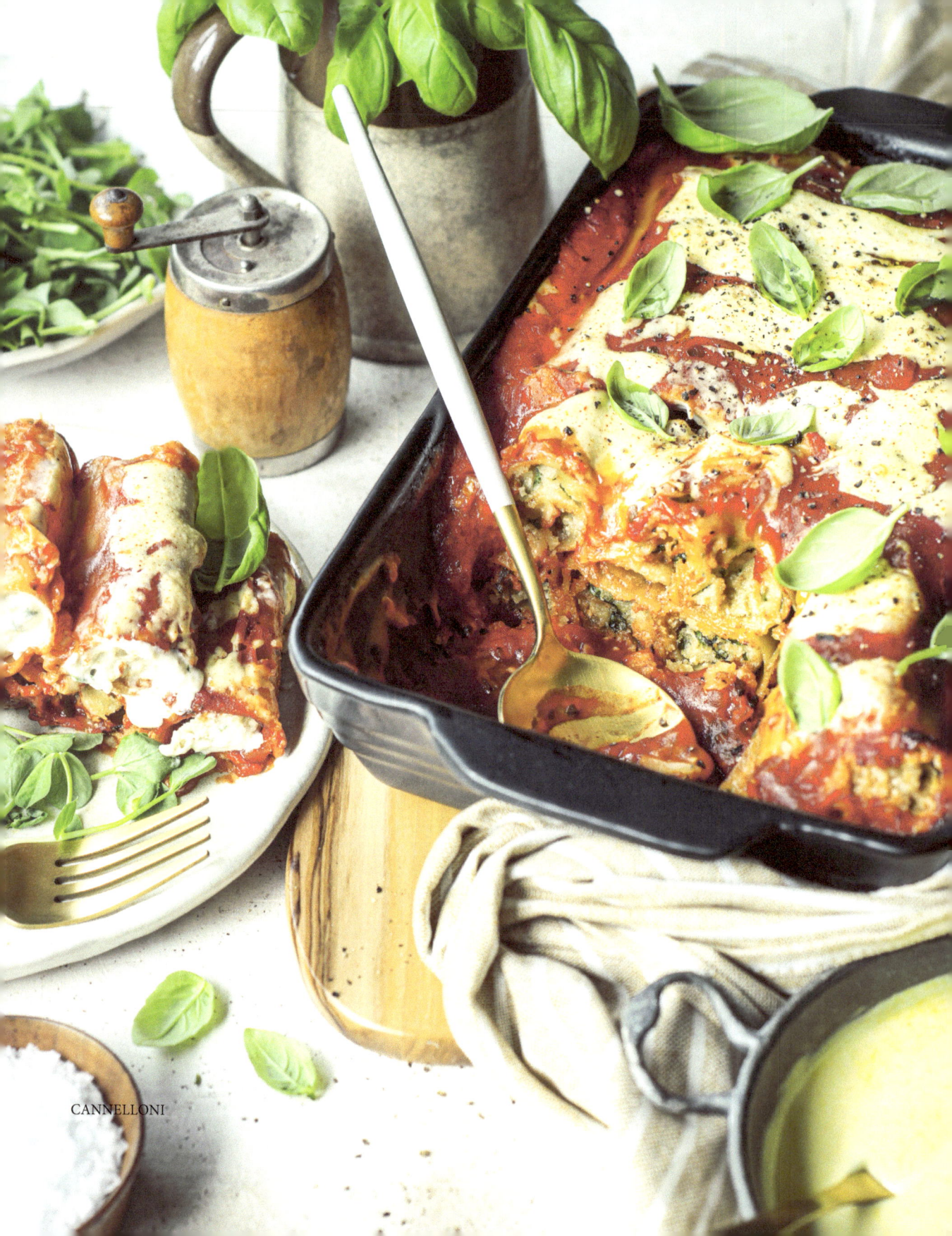

CANNELLONI

CANNELLONI

This is a classic dish my family would often make at home, which is why I was so pleased with just how much I loved this plant-based version. It's warming, hearty and so comforting, I hope you all love it as much as I do.

Ingredients
1x 250g pack Cannelloni pasta
Classic tomato pasta sauce (see 'sauces' for ingredients and amount on page 126)

Filling
500g cashews
3 tsp onion powder
3 tsp paprika
10 tbsp nutritional yeast
2 tsp soy sauce
1 cup oat milk
Salt pepper
150g Spinach

Béchamel sauce
1 cup oat milk
1 tbsp plain flour (or gluten free flour), + extra to add more if needed
½ cup nutritional yeast
Sprinkle paprika
Salt, Pepper

STEP 1
First make the pasta sauce, once cooked, cover and leave to one side. Then in a separate saucepan, add all the béchamel sauce ingredients and whisk well to remove any lumps. Bring sauce to the boil and let simmer, adding more flour if necessary for thickness (it should be relatively thick). Cook for 3–4 minutes then cover with lid.

STEP 2
Add all of the filling ingredients into a blender except the spinach and blend well. Then stir in the spinach to the mixture. Save any extra filling.

STEP 3
Cover the base of the baking tray with some of the tomato sauce to prevent sticking. Then begin to fill the cannelloni with the filling and place onto the baking tray. Continue until the tray is full.

STEP 4
Pour tomato sauce on top of cannelloni, making sure it's completely covered including the sides. Then add béchamel sauce on top. If you have any extra filling you can use add it on top of the béchamel sauce in dollops.

STEP 5
Place baking tray in the oven for 35–40 minutes (cover with tin foil is it begins to burn on top). Stab with a fork to check when it's done.

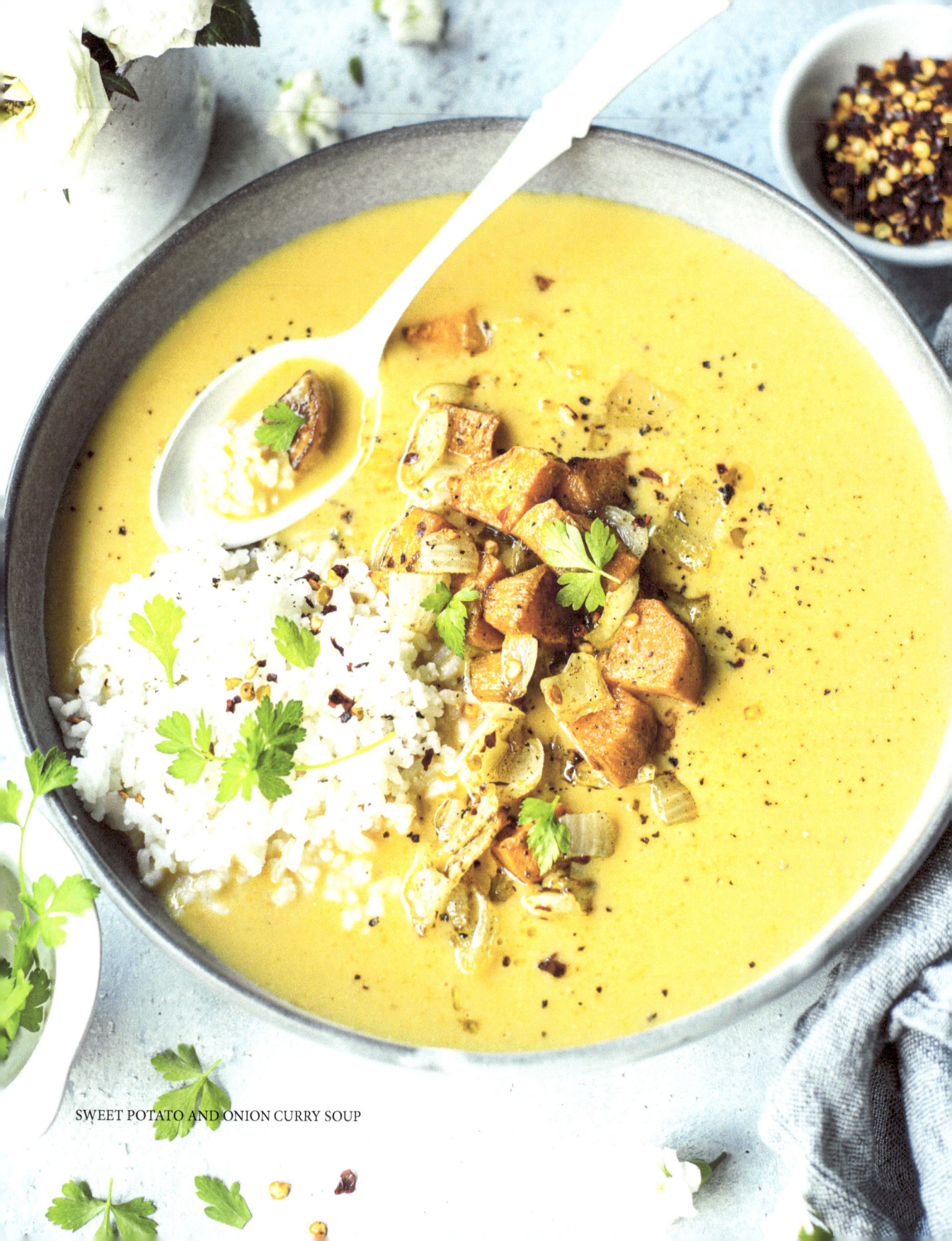

SWEET POTATO AND ONION CURRY SOUP

SWEET POTATO AND ONION CURRY SOUP

SERVES 2 PEOPLE

As far as soups go, they really don't get much better than this. The coconut milk gives the soup a fuller, creamy texture and the gentle spices from the curry powder and turmeric will warm you up from the inside making it a perfect dish for the winter months.

Ingredients

2 large roast sweet potatoes
1 onion
1 tsp cumin
Soup -
1 cup oat milk
250ml coconut milk from carton
2 cups water
1 stock cube
1 tbsp curry powder
3 tbsp nutritional yeast
1 tsp turmeric powder
2 tsp coconut sugar
Sprinkle of chili flakes (to taste)
Parsley
Salt
Serve with rice

STEP 1

Pre heat oven to 180 degrees. Peel and dice sweet potato into bitesize chunks (not too small, they shrink when cooked). Also cut the onion into large bitesize chunks. Add both to a baking tray and pour a little oil on top. Then sprinkle the cumin on top and mix all together. Bake for 35–40 Minutes.

STEP 2

In a saucepan add all of the soup ingredients and stir well. Bring to boil and then let simmer until the stock cube has dissolved. You can add more water if necessary or cook for longer to thicken.

STEP 3

Once the potato and onion are ready take out of the oven and place into the soup bowls. Then pour the soup on top.

Curry powder is a mix of different spices such as, turmeric, chili powder, coriander, ground cumin, ginger and pepper. Together this mix provides a burst of antioxidants and has powerful anti-inflammatory affects.

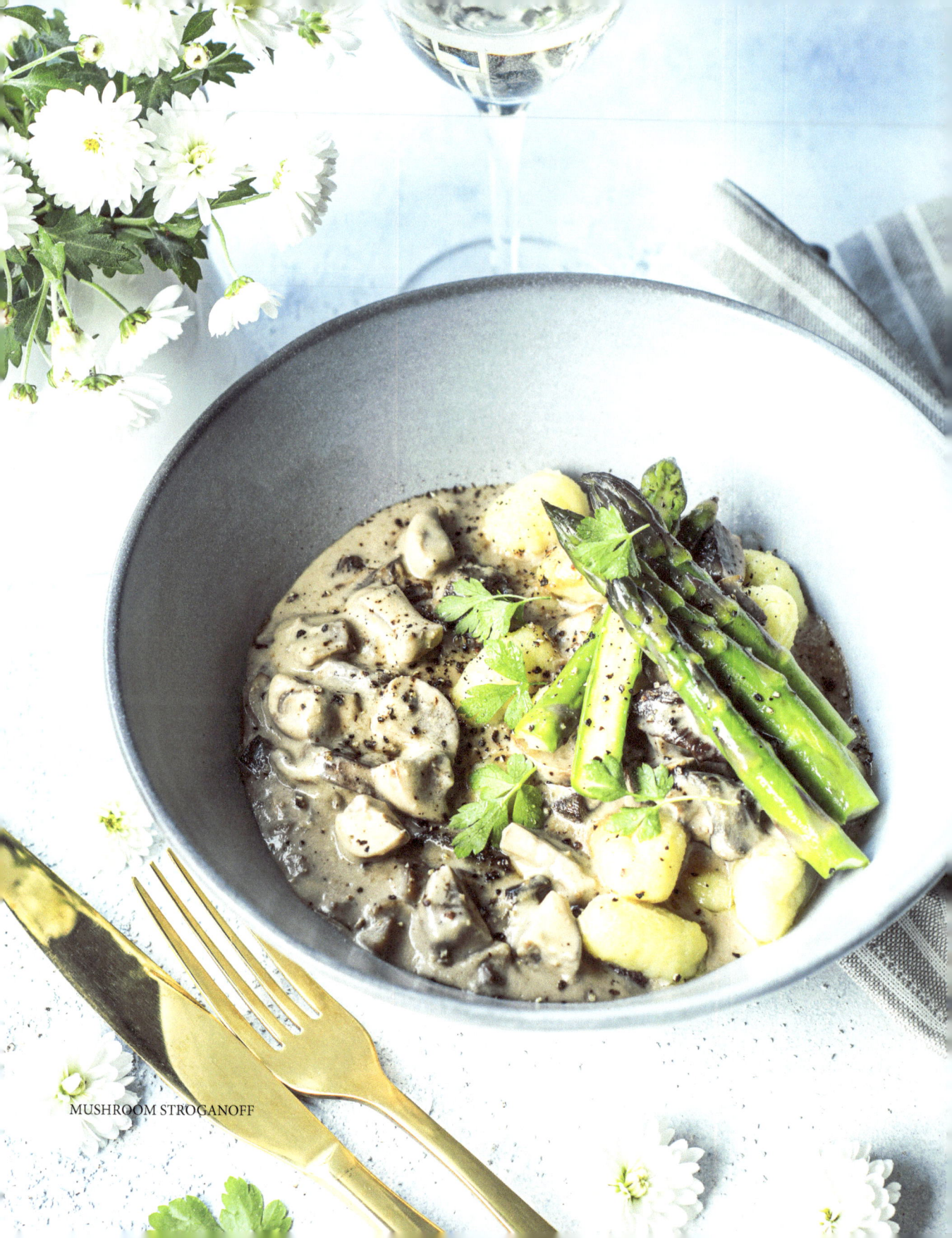

MUSHROOM STROGANOFF

MUSHROOM STROGANOFF

This is such a lovely feel-good dish and it's always a favourite. I like to serve it with gnocchi and asparagus however, it can also be served with rice or as a pasta sauce.

Ingredients

Sauce
1 large onion
1 large garlic
3tbsp vegetable gravy
1 cup water
400g coconut milk
3 tbsp nutritional yeast
1 tbsp tamari
2 tbsp spelt flour
½ tsp brown rice miso
4 tbsp mushroom water
250g chestnut or button mushrooms
50g soaked dried porcini
Serve with handful asparagus and gnocchi

STEP 1
Chop onion and garlic and fry lightly on medium heat until cooked. In a cup mix the gravy granules with the boiling water. Place the onions, garlic and gravy into a blender with all of the other sauce ingredients and blend until thoroughly mixed.

STEP 2
Wash and chop up fresh mushrooms, drain the soaked mushrooms and Sautee all together in a frying pan for 5–7 minutes until cooked. Then pour the sauce on top, bring to boil and let simmer for 5–10 minutes.

STEP 3
In a separate pan, sauté the asparagus and gnocchi until cooked.

STEP 4
Stir the stroganoff and serve on to plates along with the gnocchi and asparagus.

Mushrooms are one of the few plant-based sources of vitamin D. They also contain a special type of soluble fibre called beta-glucan. This compound works to activate parts of your immune system and helps fight off infections and can even prevent the growth of tumours. Eat your mushrooms!

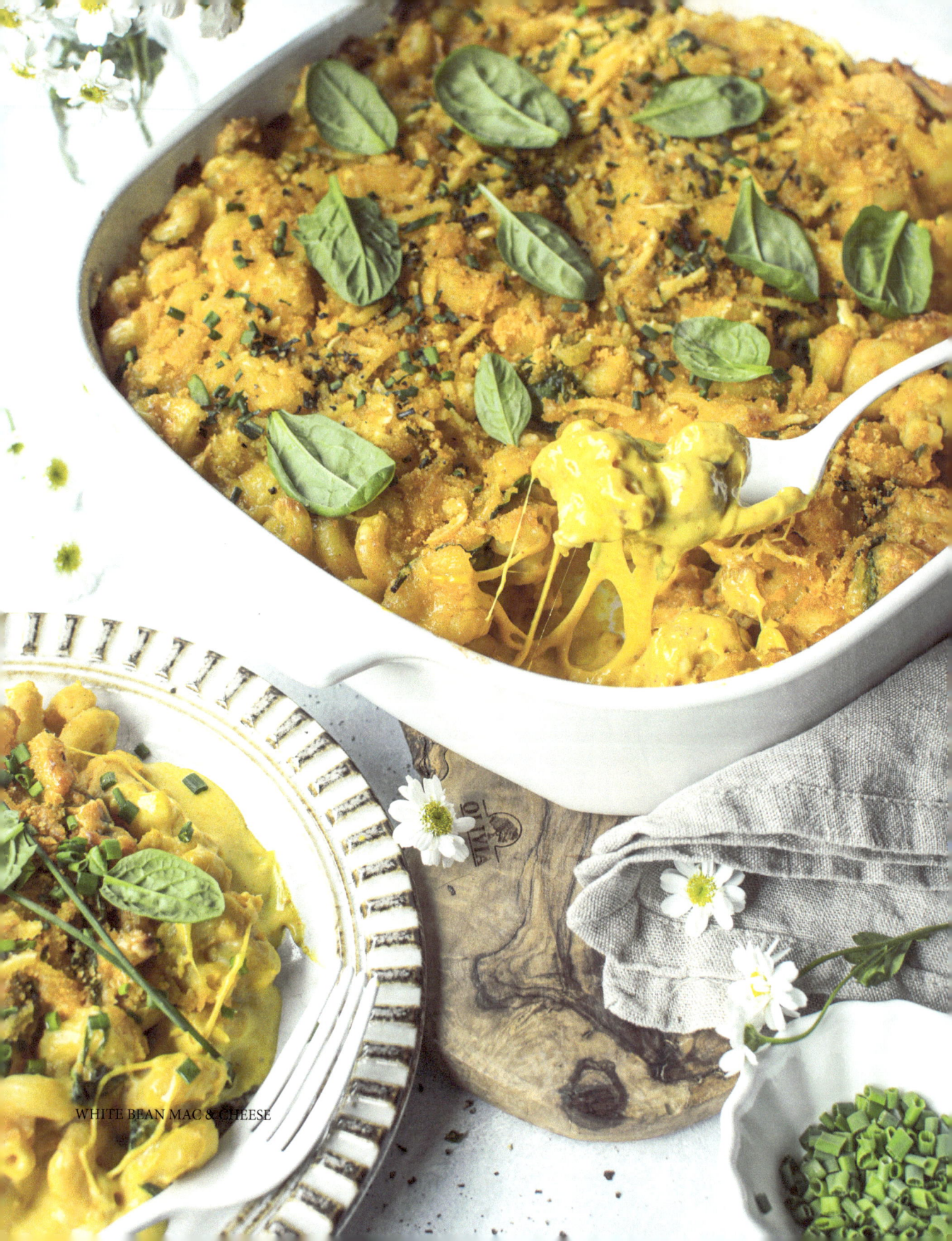

WHITE BEAN MAC & CHEESE

WHITE BEAN MAC & CHEESE

SERVES 4–5 PEOPLE

I love reinventing these classic comfort foods and adding a nutritious spin. The white beans are a great way of adding protein and fibre, and using a thicker milk like coconut or oat, it keeps the delicious creamy texture that Mac & Cheese so famous for.

Ingredients
400g white beans
1 large onion
2½ cups plant-based milk (I prefer coconut or oat)
1 cup water
1 cup nutritional yeast
1tsp paprika
Pinch turmeric for colour
Salt and pepper
450g pack macaroni pasta
2 large handfuls spinach

Topping
Vegan cheese
Breadcrumbs
Chives
(Baking tin 25x25cm)

STEP 1
Preheat oven to 180 degrees. Chop and sauté onion in frying pan. While onions cook drain beans. Then add both to a blender and blend until smooth.

STEP 2
Add all the rest of the ingredients to the blender and blend until thoroughly mixed.

STEP 3
Pour pasta into baking tray until its ¾ full, then pour the mixture on top so the macaroni is covered. Stir in spinach.

STEP 4
Cover top with your favourite plant-based cheese (shop brought or you can also use the liquid cheese or cashew cheese recipe in this book). Cover the top evenly with breadcrumbs.

STEP 5
Cover baking tray with tin foil and place in oven for 30 minutes. After that, remove tin foil and then place back inside for a further 10–15 to brown to top slightly.

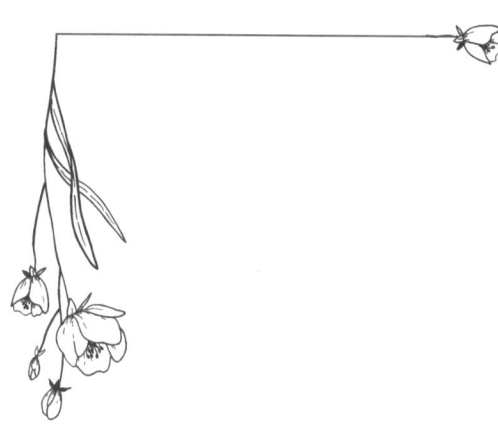

I give myself permission to eat

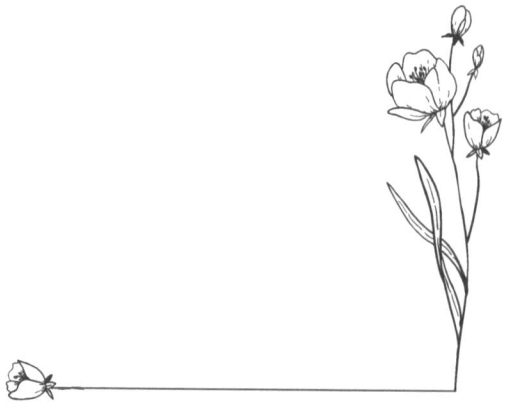

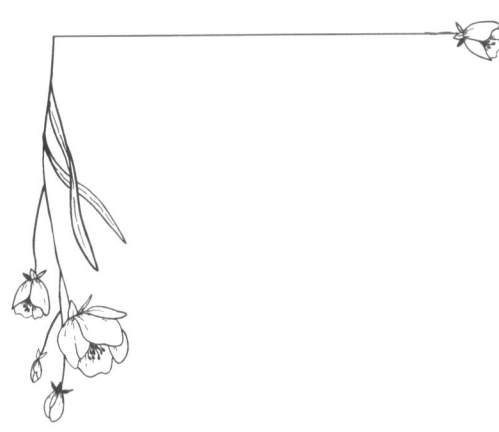

I feel good about my body today

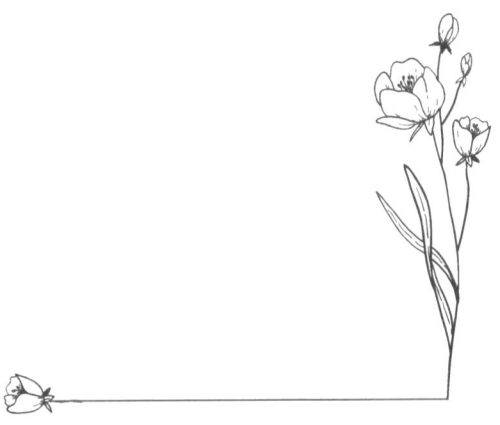

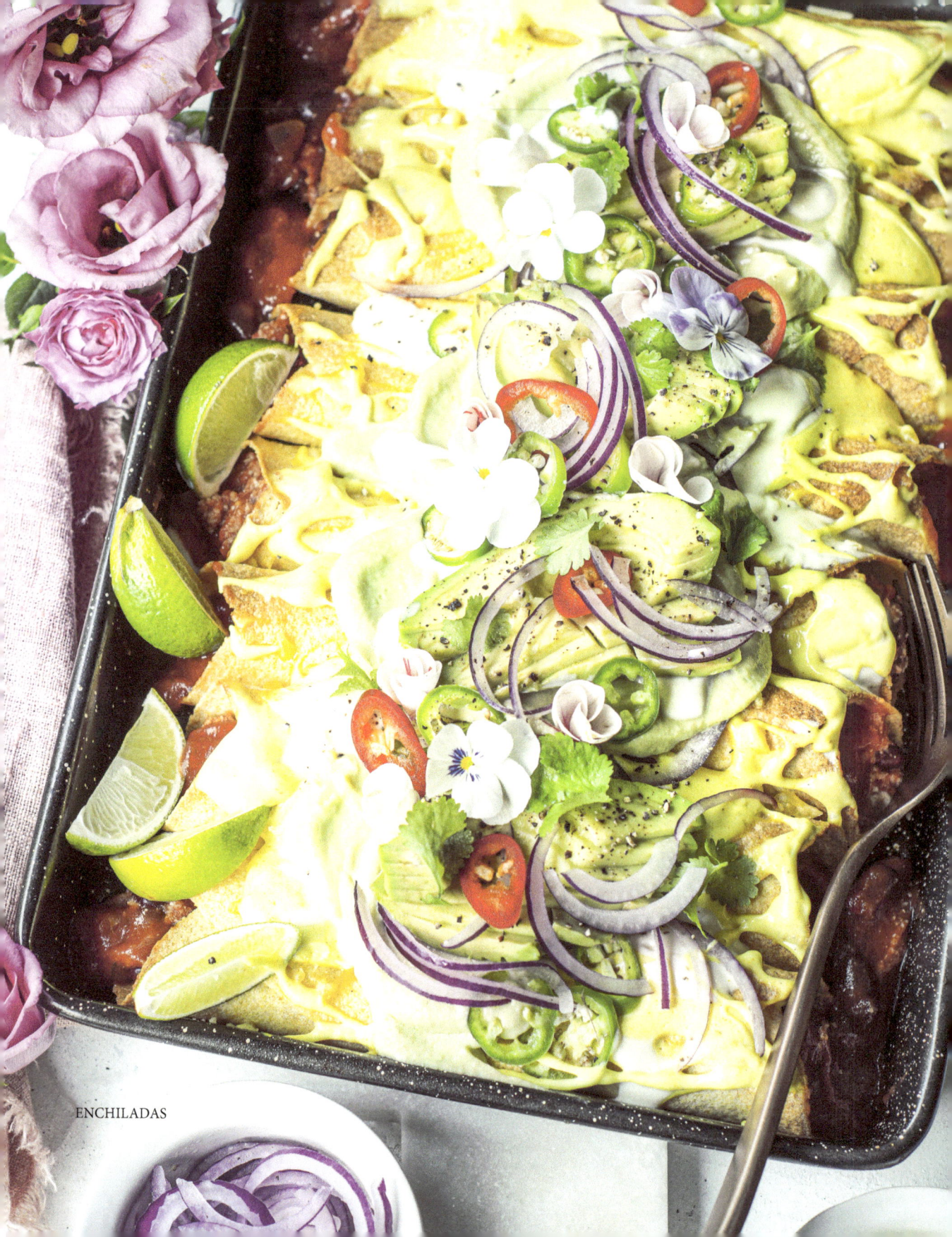

ENCHILADAS

ENCHILADAS

These enchiladas are just so yummy, not to mention a great source of plant-based protein. Perfect to eat on their own as a main meal or serve with a side of brown rice.

Ingredients

Filling
1 large onion
1 garlic
1 400g tin black or kidney beans
1 tin 400g chopped tomatoes
Sprinkle chili flakes
6 small to medium wraps (I used gluten free)

Topping
Vegan cheese
Avocado cream (see page 123)
Soy yogurt
Red onions
Chili peppers (optional)

STEP 1
Preheat oven to 180 degrees. Chop up and fry the garlic and onion for 3–5 minutes, then rinse and add the kidney beans. Cook the beans for about 3 minutes and then add the tinned tomatoes, chili flakes, salt and pepper. Bring to boil and then let simmer for 30–40 minutes.

STEP 2
Once the filling tastes ready, place about 3 tbsp of filling inside the wrap and roll it up to close, then place in baking tray. Repeat until tray is full.

STEP 3
Cover the top of the enchiladas with your favourite plant–based cheese (can use a cheese from this book, if you use the liquid cheese I recommend adding on top after cooked). Place in the oven for 15–20 minutes.

STEP 4
Remove tray from oven and top enchiladas with avocado cream, soy yogurt and red onion and chillis if using.

When we cook tomatos a chemical called lycopene increases. Lycopene is a potent antioxidant and has been proven to prevent cell damage and have anti–cancer properties.

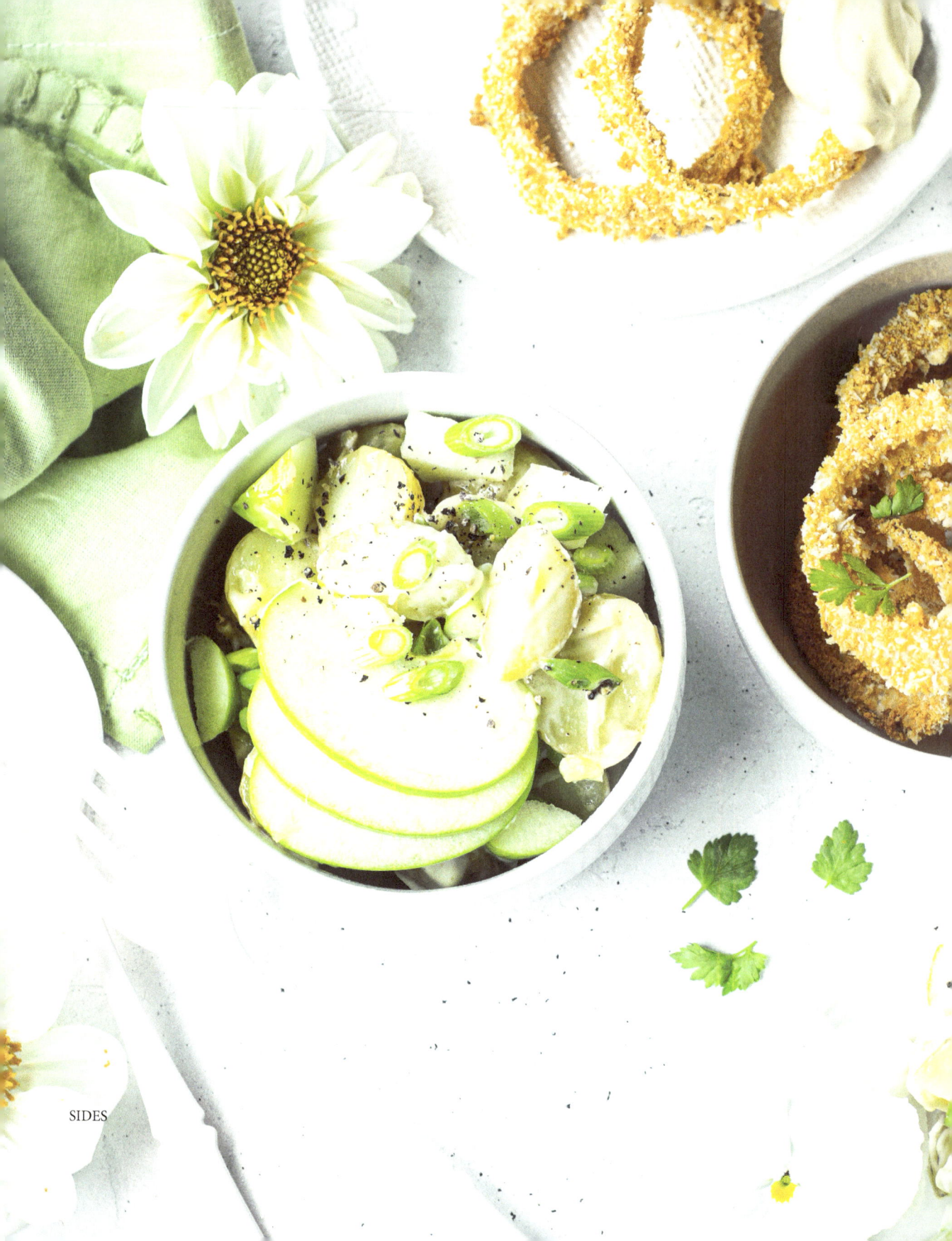

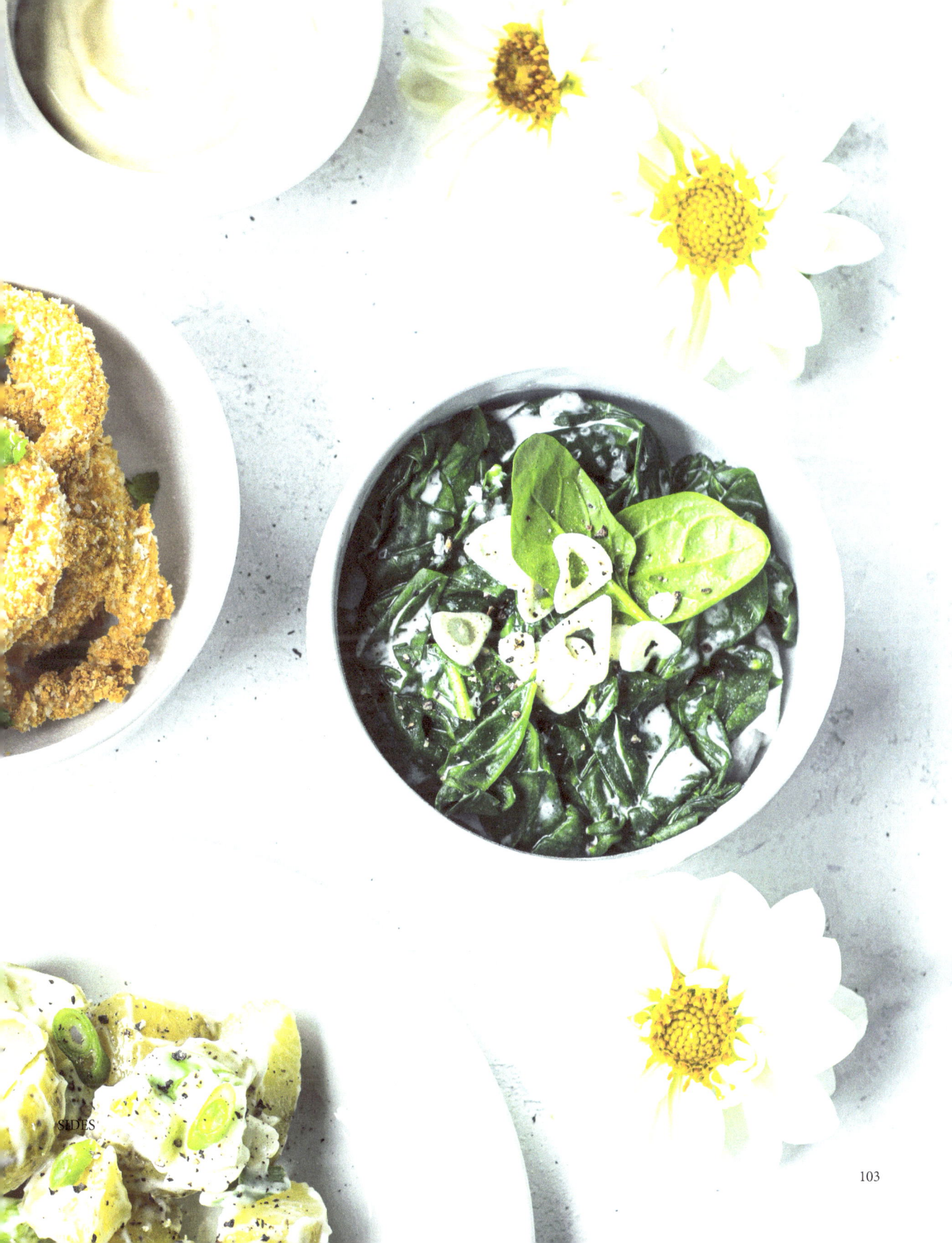

SIDES

Side dishes really complete any meal. Weather it's some creamy spinach on the side of your roast dinner, a potato salad with your veggie burger at a barbeque or some onion rings on the dinner table for everyone to share, we all love them! So enjoy these three super easy yet super tasty side dishes.

CREAMY SPINACH

SERVES 2 PEOPLE

Ingredients
150g fresh baby spinach
6 tbsp coconut milk from can or carton
1 garlic
Salt

STEP 1
Fill up kettle and boil. While the kettle is boiling was the spinach. Then in a pan, add the spinach and pour boiling water on top till the spinach wilts. If it has not fully wilted then apply heat until it has done so. Once spinach has wilted, drain well to remove any excess water.

STEP 2
Place spinach in a bowl, add salt, chop up garlic and add. Open the coconut milk (do not shake beforehand), and add the table spoons from the white layer that usually sits on top.

STEP 3
Stir well and serve.

POTATO SALAD

Ingredients
Baby potatoes
Spring onions
Green apple

Dressing
200g tofu
2 tbsp cashew butter
¼ tsp mustard Dijon
Squeeze lemon
1tsp coconut sugar
Salt
pepper

STEP 1
In a saucepan, boil potatoes until they're soft enough to stab.

STEP 2
In a blender while potatoes are cooking, add all the dressing ingredients and blend until thoroughly mixed.

STEP 3
Chop up the apple and onions and place in bowl. When the potatoes are ready, drain and chop them up into bite size pieces and add them to the same bowl.

STEP 4
Add the dressing, mix well and serve.

ONION RINGS

Ingredients
1 cup oat milk
3 tbsp plain flour
1 tbsp melted coconut oil
3–4 onions
1 cup breadcrumbs
Salt
Pepper
Parsley

STEP 1
Preheat oven to 180 degrees. Combine the oat milk, flour and coconut oil into a bowl and whisk till smooth. Then in a separate bowl combine the breadcrumbs, salt, pepper and parsley.

STEP 2
Slice the onion and separate to make rings. Then dip the onion first into the wet mix, make sure it's thoroughly covered, and then into the breadcrumbs. Place on a baking tray.

STEP 3
Once the baking tray is full, place it into the oven for around 30 minutes.

STEP 4
Serve with vegan mayonnaise (see page 127) or liquid cheese sauce (see page 121).

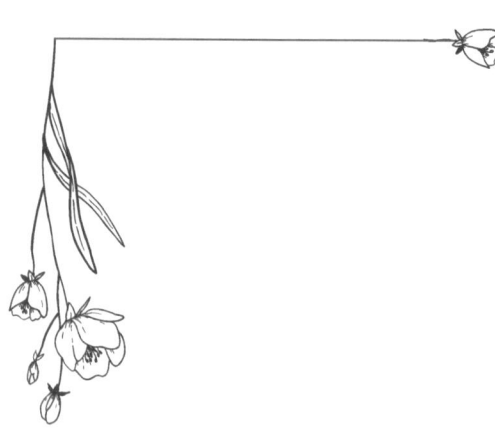

I always listen to what my body is telling me

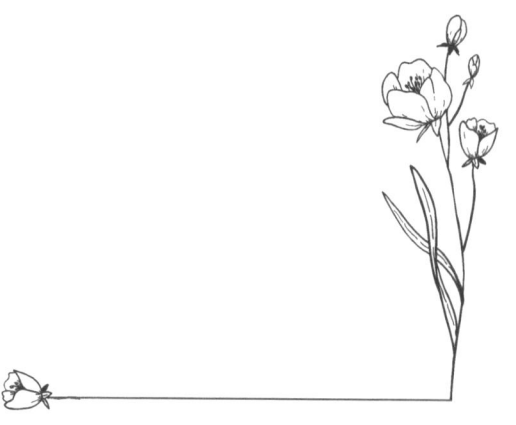

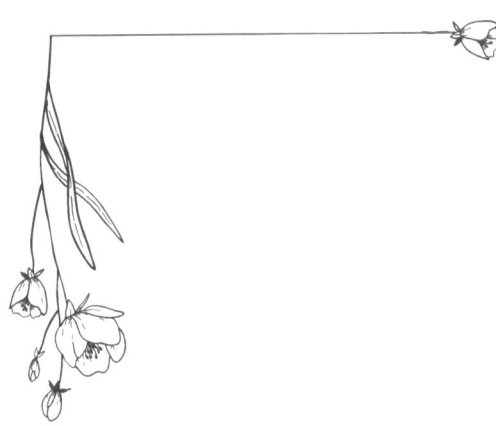

I have unlimited energy

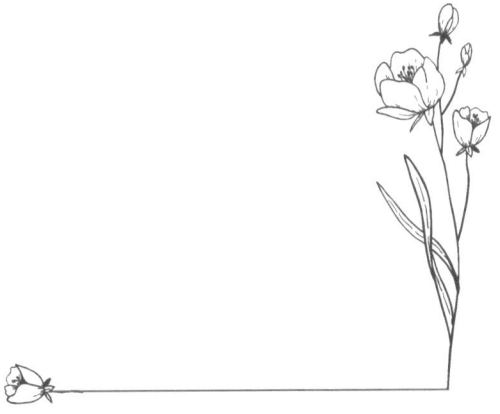

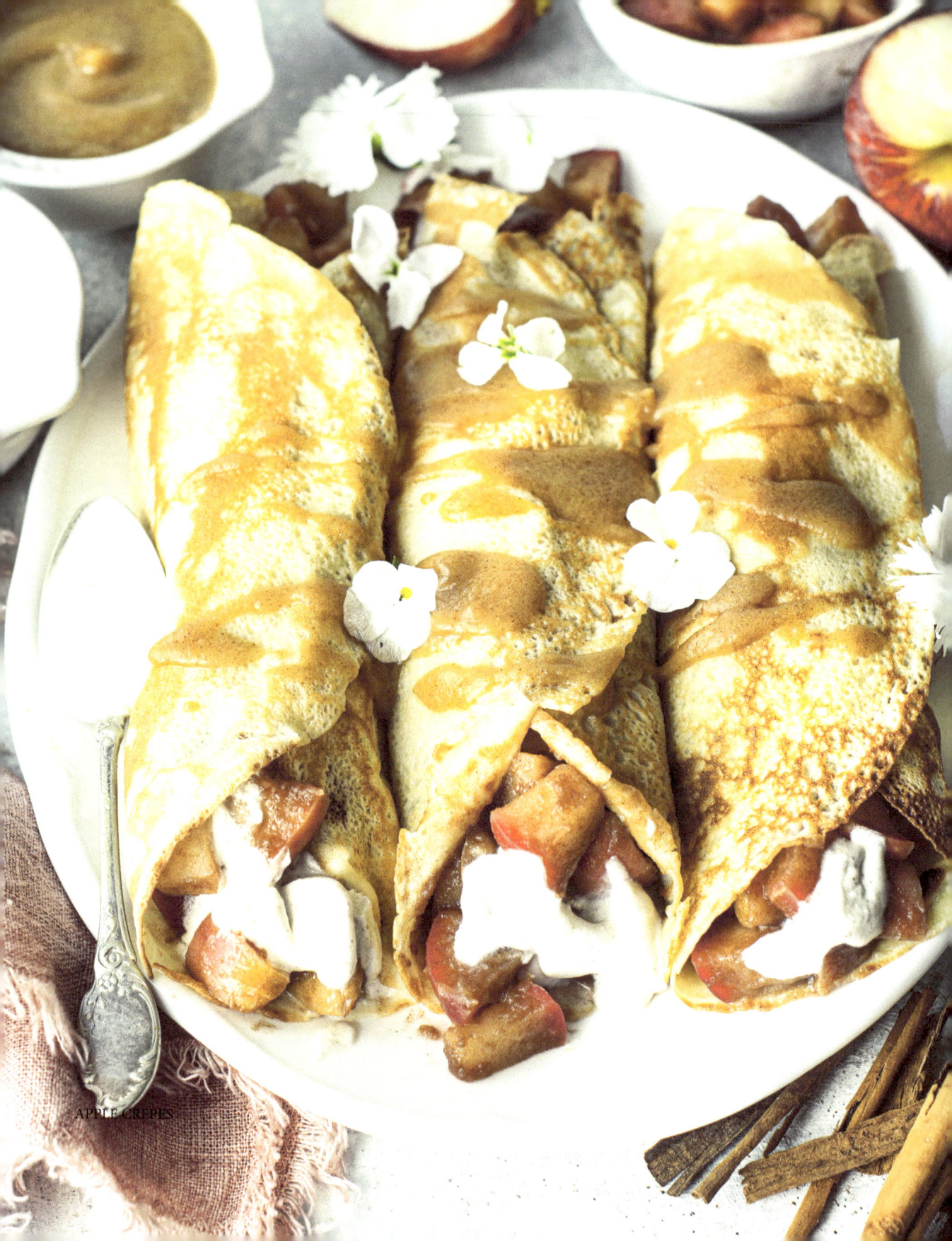

APPLE CREPES

DESERTS

This is one of my favourite sweet recipes in the book because it really just makes you feel good. The apple and cinnamon together naturally give it a warm, indulgent feeling, which makes it perfect for when you're just wanting to cosy up on the sofa with something sweet.

APPLE CREPES

Ingredients
160 g spelt flour
2 tbsp maple syrup
300ml plant-based milk (I use oat milk)
1 tbsp coconut oil

Apple filling
3 large red sweet apples
3 tbsp water
1 tsp cinnamon
Stir in 2 tbsp apple purée

Date paste
6 dates
2 tbsp coconut milk
Salt

STEP 1
Wash and chop apples into small bite size pieces and place into saucepan. Add the water and cinnamon and stir. Put on a medium heat and cover with lid, stirring occasionally. Turn the heat down a bit of they are sizzling too much to avoid burning. Cook until soft.

STEP 2
Whisk together all of the pancake ingredients. In a frying pan heat up a small amount of coconut oil, then add a ladle of pancake mix. Allow to cook and then flip over to cook to other side. Repeat until all of the mixture is used up.

STEP 3
In a blender combine all of the date paste ingredients and blend to form a paste.

STEP 4
Once apples have finished cooking, stir in the apple sauce. Then begin to fill the pancakes with the date paste and the apple filling.

STEP 5
Serve with cinnamon coconut cream (see page 123)

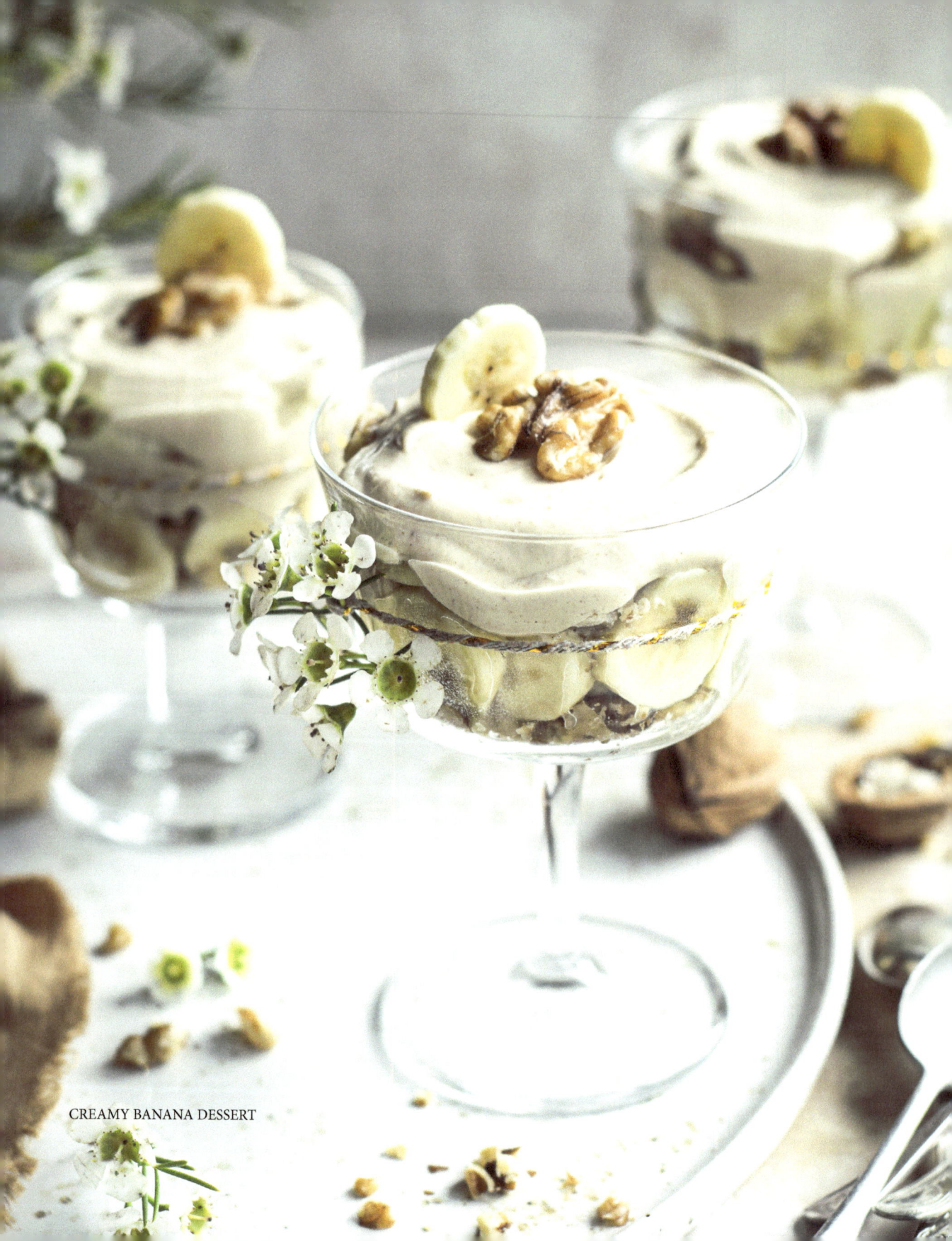

CREAMY BANANA DESSERT

CREAMY BANANA DESSERT

Served chilled, it's packed with protein and the tofu gives it a very light mousse-like texture, which makes it a great dessert or even snack for the summer months. I love how simple this recipe is, it really could not be easier to make.

Ingredients
Peanut butter tofu cream (see page 123)
1 large chopped banana
A handful of crushed walnuts

STEP 1
In a dessert glass, first add some banana, then some walnuts, then peanut butter tofu cream. Keep layering until glass it full. Top with nuts and banana.

Tofu is great because it contains all 9 amino acids. Amino acids are the building blocks for proteins and are essential for process such as cell building. It also contains calcium, iron, magnesium and zinc.

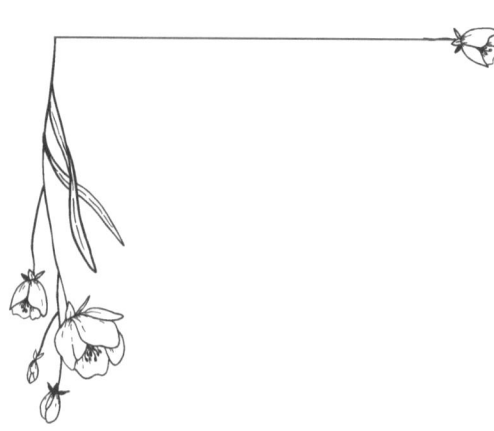

I appreciate my body and all the hard work it does for me

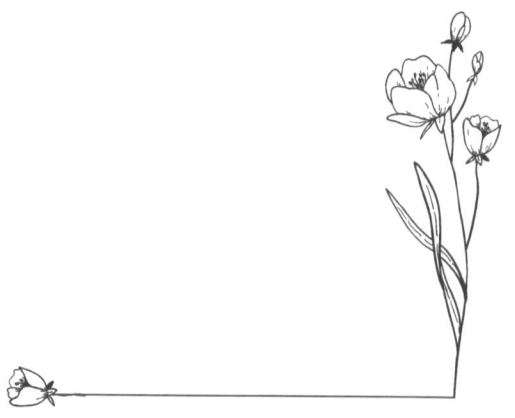

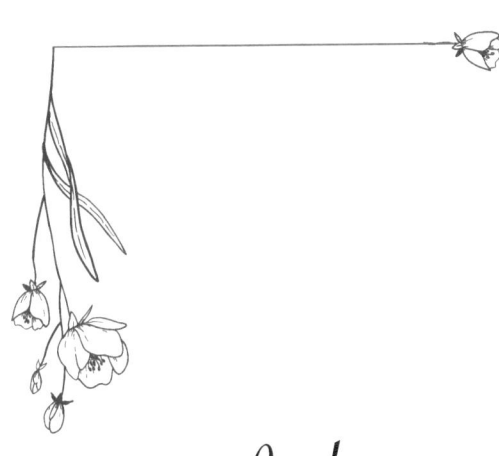

I choose to let go of all my
negative feelings and fill myself
with love.

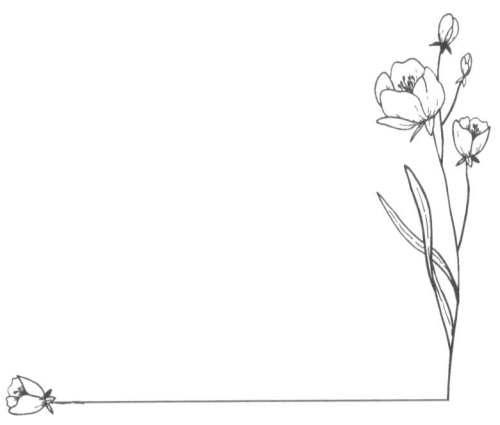

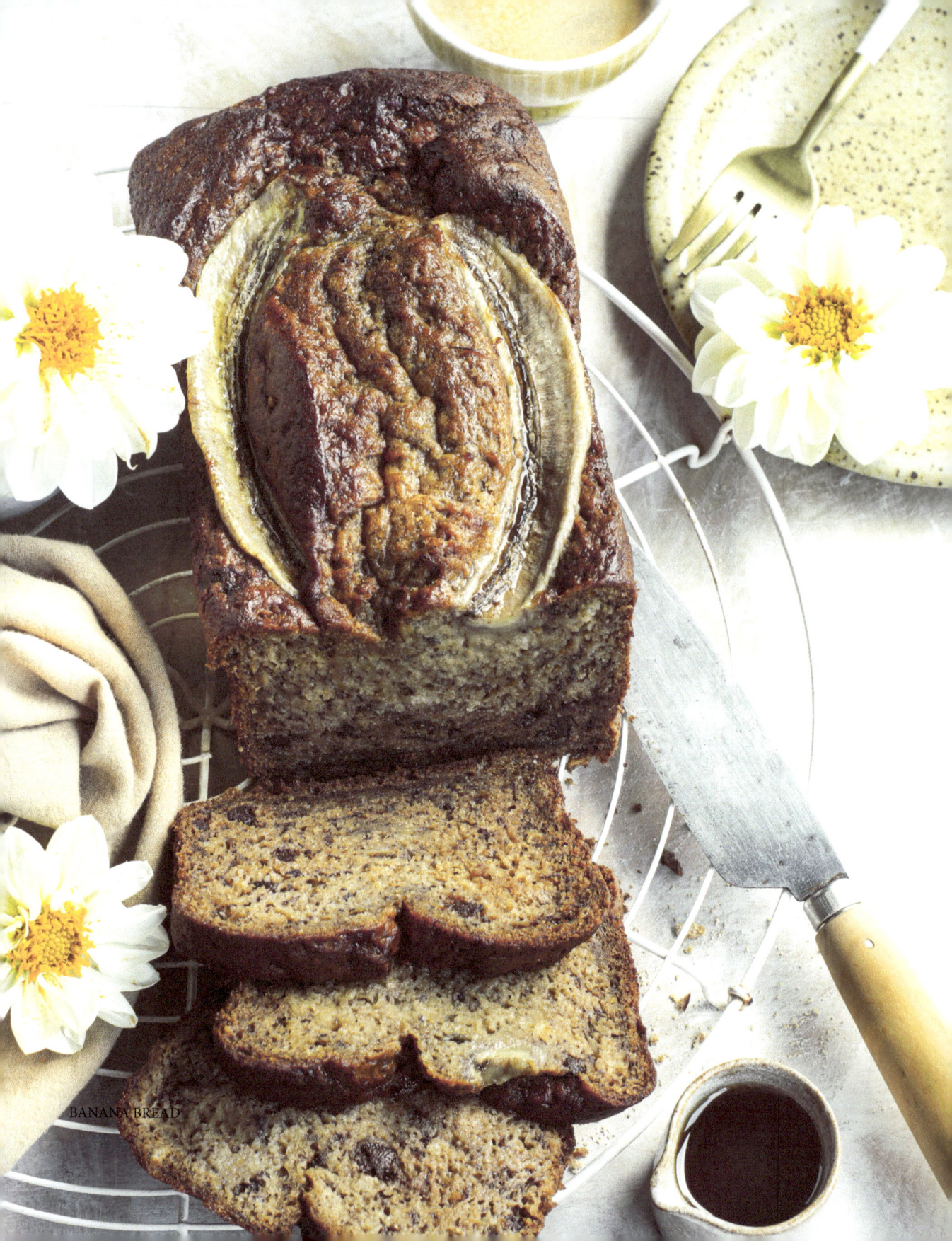

BANANA BREAD

BANANA BREAD

This is a classic recipe in our house, I make it all the time and it's loved by everyone. The bananas and olive oil give the bread a lovely moist texture. This recipe is pretty versatile as the bread isn't too sweet, making it a great on the go breakfast. Snack on it as it is, or toast it and top it with nut butter and cream and enjoy it as a dessert.

Ingredients

2 cups spelt flour
1 cup coconut sugar
3 tsp baking powder
1 vanilla pod
¼ cup olive oil
¼ cup water
4 mashed bananas
Vegan chocolate chips (optional)
Extra banana for decoration (optional)
Bake for 35 mins at 180 degrees
(Baking tin 25cm)

STEP 1
Preheat oven to 180 degrees. In a mixing bowl combine all the ingredients except the chocolate chips and whisk. Then stir in the chocolate chips if using.

STEP 2
Line a small bread tin with baking paper and pour in the cake mixture. If using the extra banana then peel it and cut it in half long ways (as shown on the cake in picture). Lay each piece on top of the cake and place in oven for 30–35 minutes.

STEP 3
Test the cake is ready by placing a knife directly in the middle and see if it comes out clean. If so, take the cake out of the oven and let it stand in the tin for minimum 20 minutes.

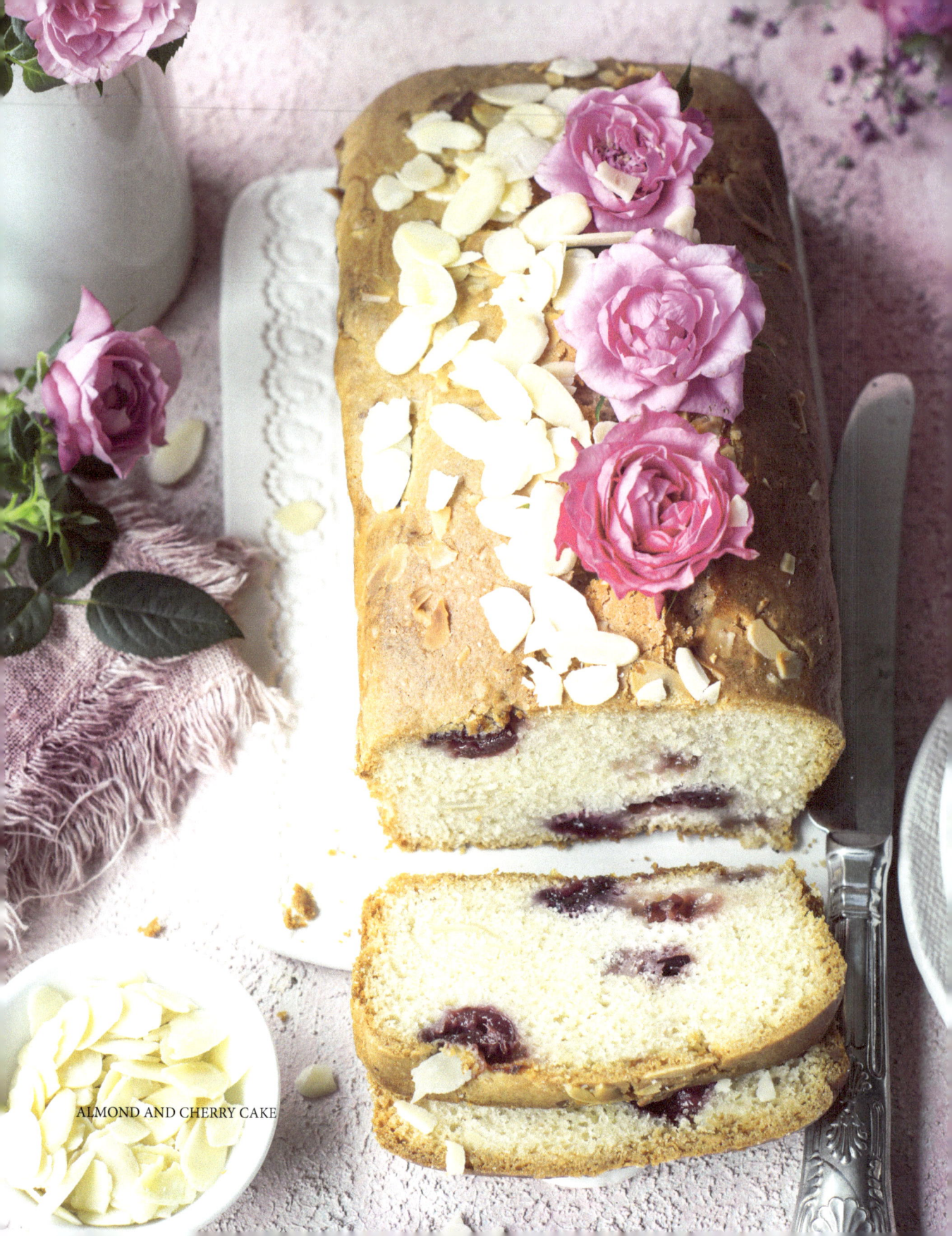

ALMOND AND CHERRY CAKE

ALMOND AND CHERRY CAKE

This sweet, moist, delicious cherry and almond cake always gives me a summery feeling. The sweet fruitiness of the cherries and the light nutty flavours of the shaved almonds and coconut milk all complement each other so well. I tend to eat the cake just like this as it is, but feel free top with some almond or cashew butter.

Ingredients

250g spelt flour
3tsp baking powder
150ml coconut milk
6 tbsp coconut oil
150ml maple syrup
2 vanilla pods
Big handful shaved almonds
200g fresh cherries
Bake 45 minutes (knife test is clear)
Serve with cherries fresh for deco
(Baking tin 25–13cm)

STEP 1

Preheat oven to 180 degrees. Combine all of the ingredients except the cherries and almonds in a mixing bowl and whisk together well. Then stir in the cherries and almond, saving some almonds to place on top later.

STEP 2

Line a small bread tin with greaseproof paper and pour in the cake mixture. Sprinkle the rest of the almond shavings on top and the place in the oven. Bake for about 45 minutes.

STEP 3

Test the cake is ready by placing a knife directly in the middle and see if it comes out clean. If so, take the cake out of the oven and let it stand in the tin for minimum 20 minutes.

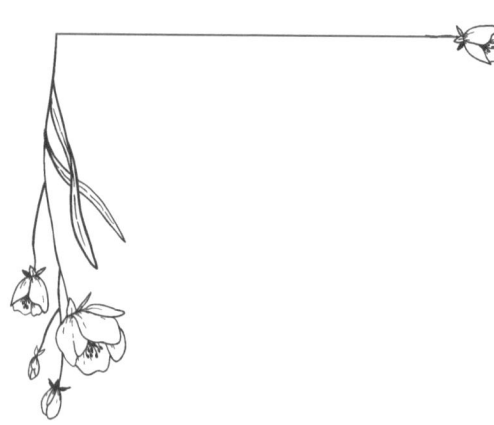

I am in tune with my body

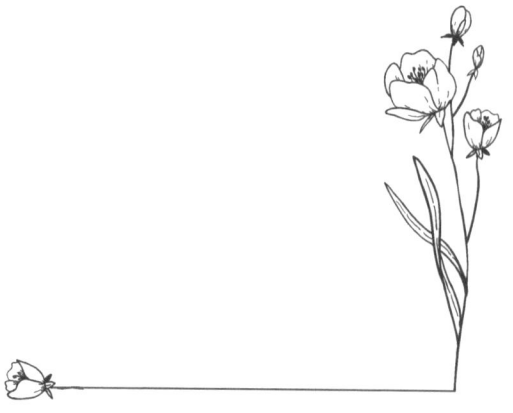

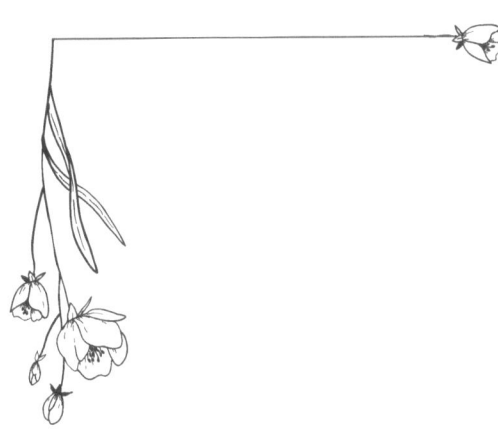

I am grateful for the abundance
of food

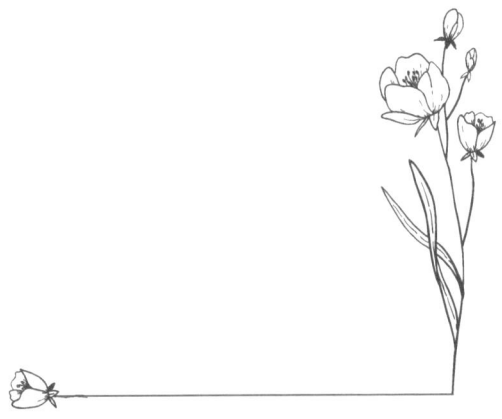

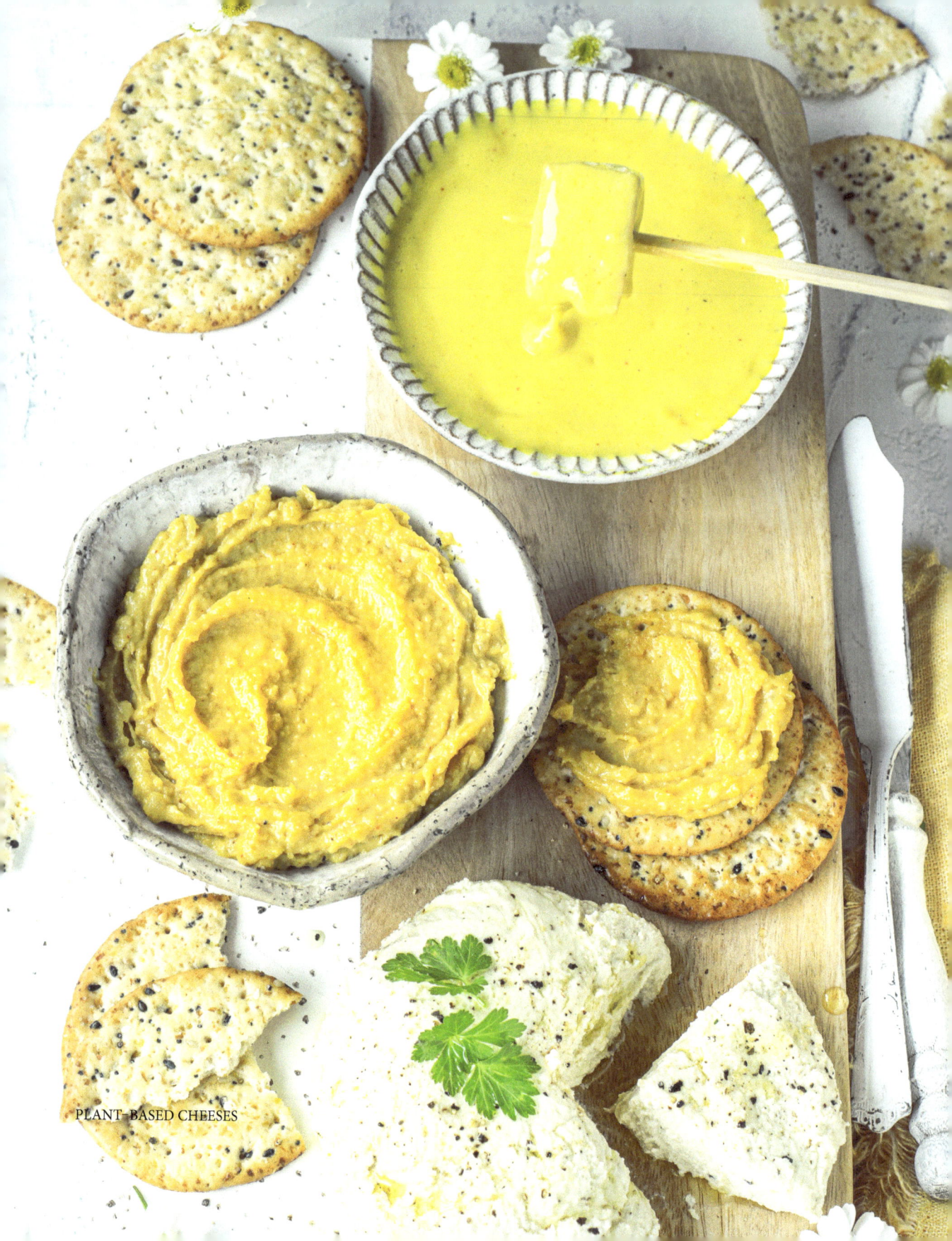

PLANT-BASED CHEESES

PLANT-BASED CHEESES

For many people cheese is the one thing that they feel would be impossible to replace. But with the right ingredients we can manage to mimic its unique flavour and use it as a healthful alternative in our favourite recipes.

TOFU RICOTTA

Enjoy on a cracker with some caramelised onion or fig topping.

Ingredients
230g hard tofu
1 tbsp Olive oil
3 tsp nutritional yeast
Squeeze lemon juice
150g soy yogurt
Salt
Top with olive oil and parsley

STEP 1
Place all ingredients in a blender and blend, keeping it a touch grainy.

STEP 2
You can either eat it like that or put in a cheese mould for the classic ricotta shape. Top with olive oil and parsley.

——————— TIP ———————

If you don't have a cheese mould you can also use a small foil pie baking tin to create a similar shape.

CASHEW CHEESE SPREAD

Spread in a sandwich, add to pasta or use as a cheesy topping.

Ingredients
200g cashews
½ cup nutritional yeast
½ tsp onion powder
1 tsp paprika
Pinch turmeric for colour
Salt

STEP 1
Add all the ingredients into a blender and blend until desired consistency.

LIQUID SAUCE CHEESE

Use this to top your favourite foods (great on nachos), use it in your sandwich or burrito, or even bake it in a lasagne.

Ingredients
250ml Ccoconut milk from carton
5 tbsp tapioca flour (add more if not thick enough)
¼ cup nutritional yeast
½ tsp onion powder
½ tsp paprika
Pinch turmeric for colour
Salt
Pepper

STEP 1
Add all the ingredients to a saucepan and whisk well until smooth.

STEP 2
Bring to boil and then simmer on a medium heat. Adding more flour it needed for thickness. Cook for about 3 minutes.

STEP 3
Adjust any flavouring to proffered taste. For example, more salt, a touch more onion powder.

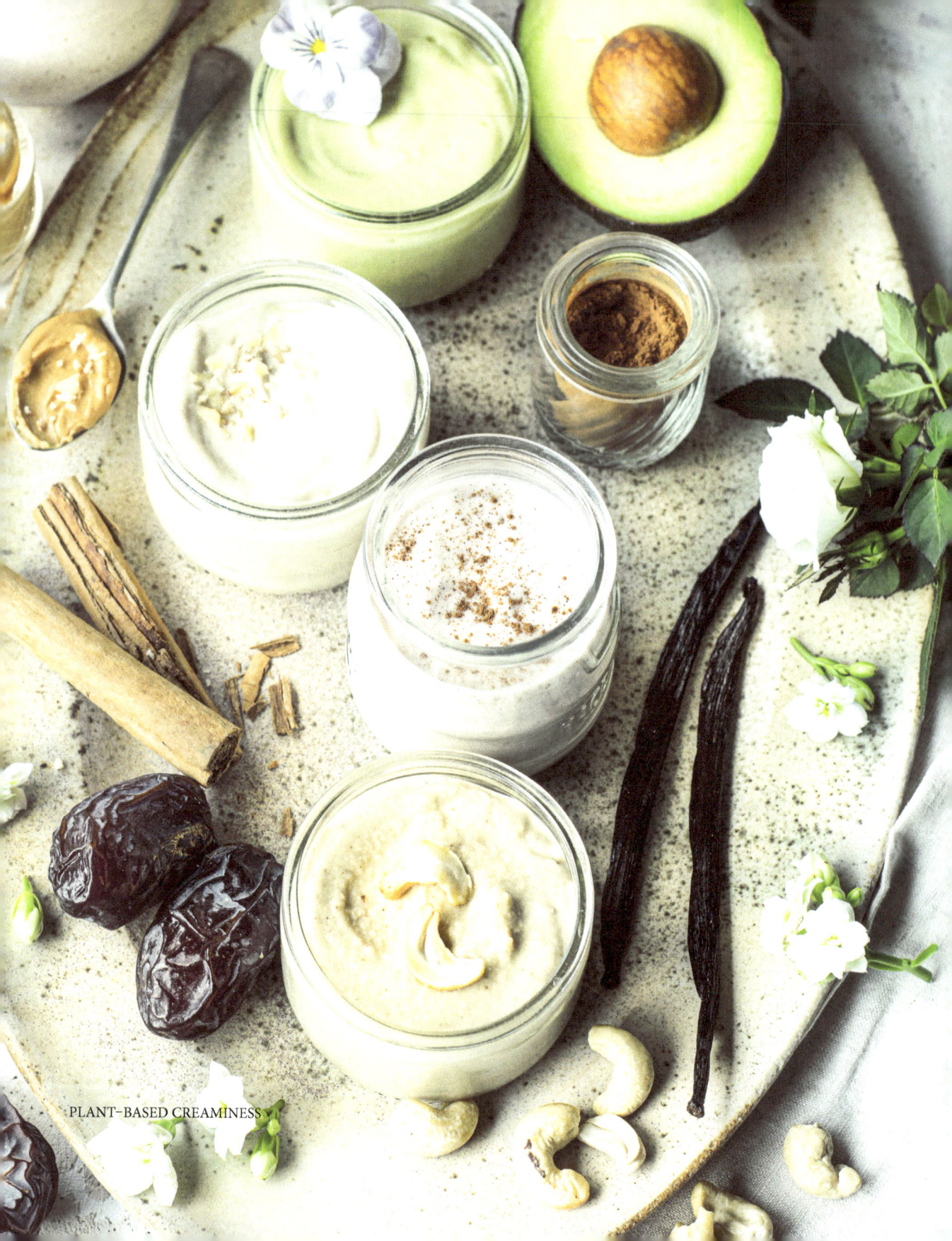

PLANT-BASED CREAMINESS

PLANT-BASED CREAMINESS

Here we have four totally different delicious options. The tofu cream is light in texture, high in protein and it's something that taste so good it might make you want to eat it out of the bowl as a 'mousse' just as it is. The cashew cream is delicious, sweeter than the tofu one, and its perfect to serve as a thick dollop on top of a cake or add more milk and pour it onto a dessert. The cinnamon cream goes amazingly with puddings like apple crumble, fruit pies, crepes and waffles. And last but not least an avocado cream, perfect for savoury dishes like enchiladas and nachos.

TOFU PEANUT BUTTER CREAM

400g silken tofu
2 heaped tbsp peanut butter
1½ tbsp maple syrup
1 vanilla pod
Small sprinkle salt

STEP 1
Pat tofu dry to remove and excess water. Then place all ingredients into a blender and blend until smooth.

CASHEW CREAM

200g cashews
2–3 dates
1 vanilla
½ cup oat milk (more for desired thickness)
Small sprinkle salt

STEP 1
Place all ingredients into a blender and blend until smooth. Add more milk for thinner consistency.

COCONUT CINNAMON CREAM

250 ml coconut cream from carton
Add 1 tsp cinnamon
1 tsp maple syrup
Adjust taste as desired

STEP 1
Shake coconut cream well, then combine all ingredients into a blender and blend. (You can also make this in a normal bowl and just stir with a spoon, but it does mix better in a blender.)

CREAMY AVOCADO

Perfect for topping enchiladas, nachos or spread in a sandwich.

1 avocado
½ cup oat milk
1 big tsp Dijon mustard
1 tbsp nutritional yeast
Salt

STEP 1
Place all ingredients into a blender and blend until smooth.

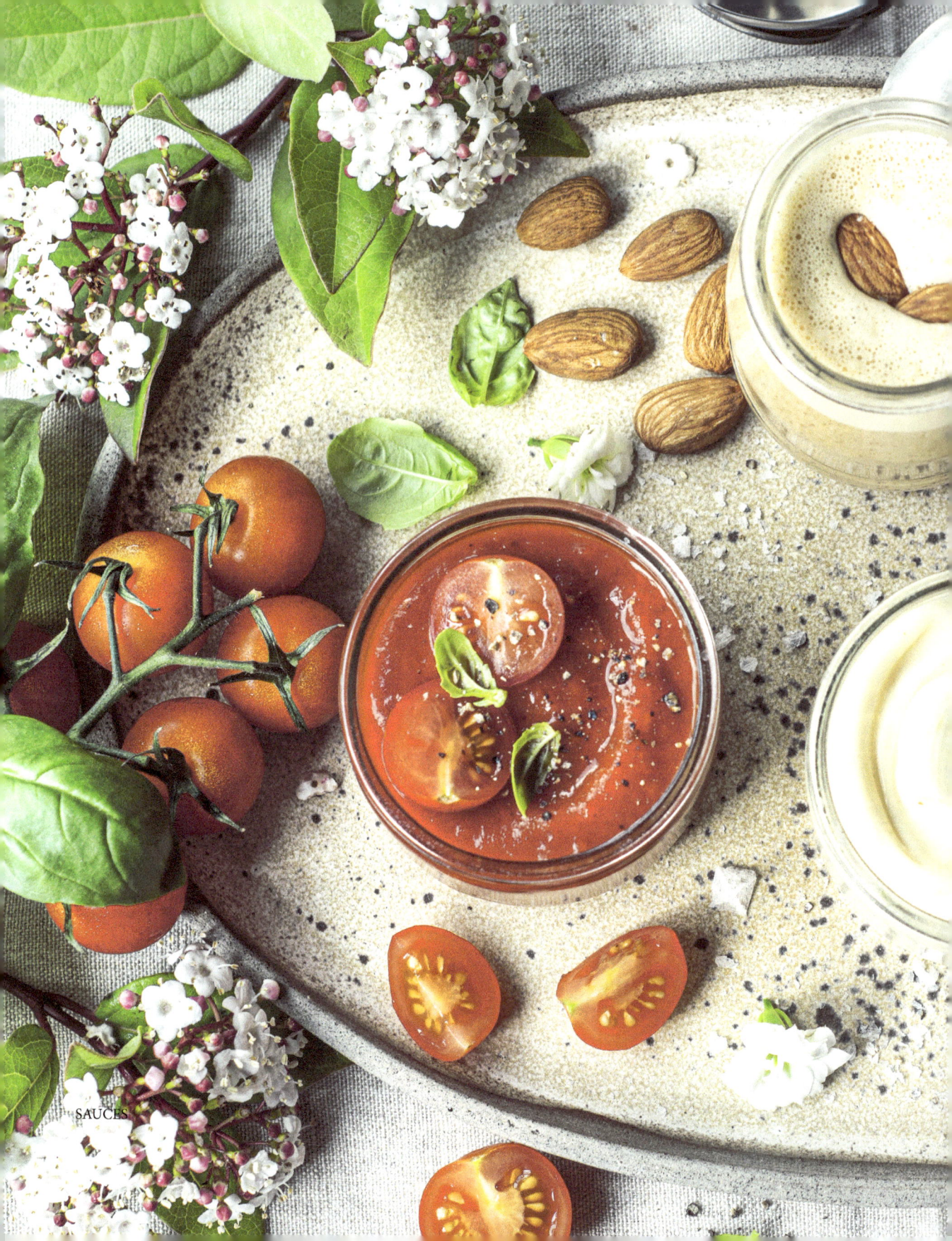

SAUCES

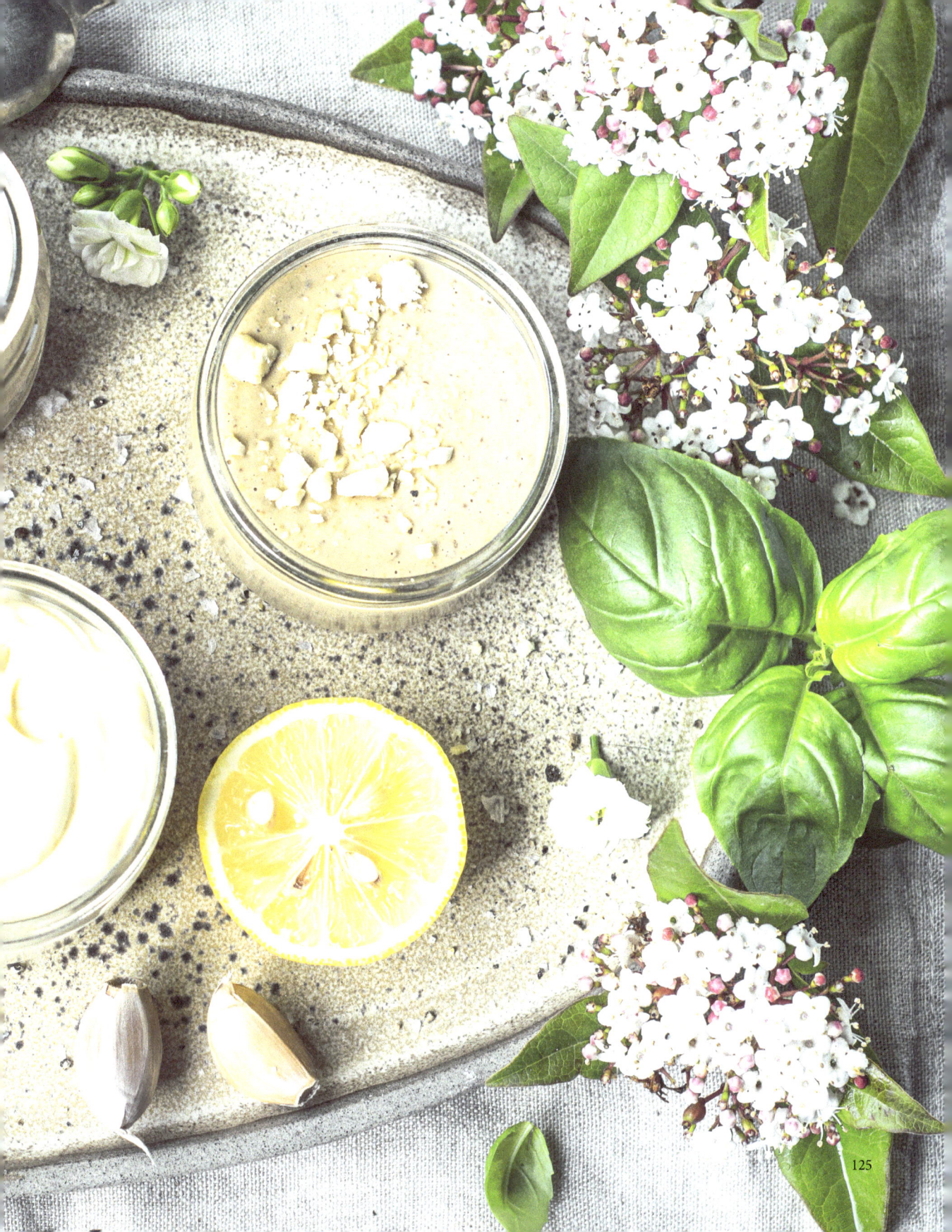

SAUCES

Every great meal out there relies on a great sauce. Pasta relies on its sauce just like roast dinners rely on the gravy, and in every great sandwich, there'll be a sauce in there somewhere too. Here is a variety of easy to make, versatile, delicious sauces.

ASIAN MISO SAUCE

Use this sauce to coat your favourite vegetables (it goes great with roasted aubergine), pour it onto a salad or use it as a dipping sauce for your spring rolls.

½ tsp Brown rice miso
½ cup oat milk
1 tbsp nutritional yeast
1 tbsp almond butter
1 tsp tamari
A few drops of rice vinegar
Sprinkle salt

STEP 1
Place all ingredients into a blender and blend until smooth.

CLASSIC TOMATO PASTA SAUCE

SERVES 1-2 PEOPLE

As it says in itss title, you can use this sauce for your pasta, however it also goes great over mixed stir–fried vegetables.

1 large onion
1 clove garlic
400g tinned tomatoes
200g water from tin
Sprinkle parsley, basil, salt and pepper

STEP 1
On a chopping board, finely dice the onion and garlic and fry on a medium heat in the saucepan for about 3–5 minutes until cooked.

STEP 2
Then add the tinned tomatoes, water and herbs and bring to boil, then simmer with lid half on for 40 mins to 1 hour, longer the better.

———— **NOTES ————
When making cannelloni or lasagne use 4 tins of tomatoes for a standard tray, and double the rest of the ingredients.

CREAMY MUSTARD SAUCE

Possibly the best addition to any sandwich out there. This sauce combines the zing flavour of the mustard with a wonderful creamy texture.

1 level tsp mustard
2 tbsp cashew butter
3–4 tbsp oat milk
1 tbsp nutritional yeast
Salt

STEP 1
Place all ingredients into a blender and blend until smooth.

GARLIC MAYONNAISE

200g silken tofu
1 roasted garlic or ¼ tsp garlic powder
1 tsp cashew butter
Squeeze lemon
Salt

STEP 1
Preheat oven to 180 degrees. Peel garlic, place in oven, lightly drizzle with olive oil and roast for 10 minutes.

STEP 2
Place all ingredients into a blender and blend until smooth.

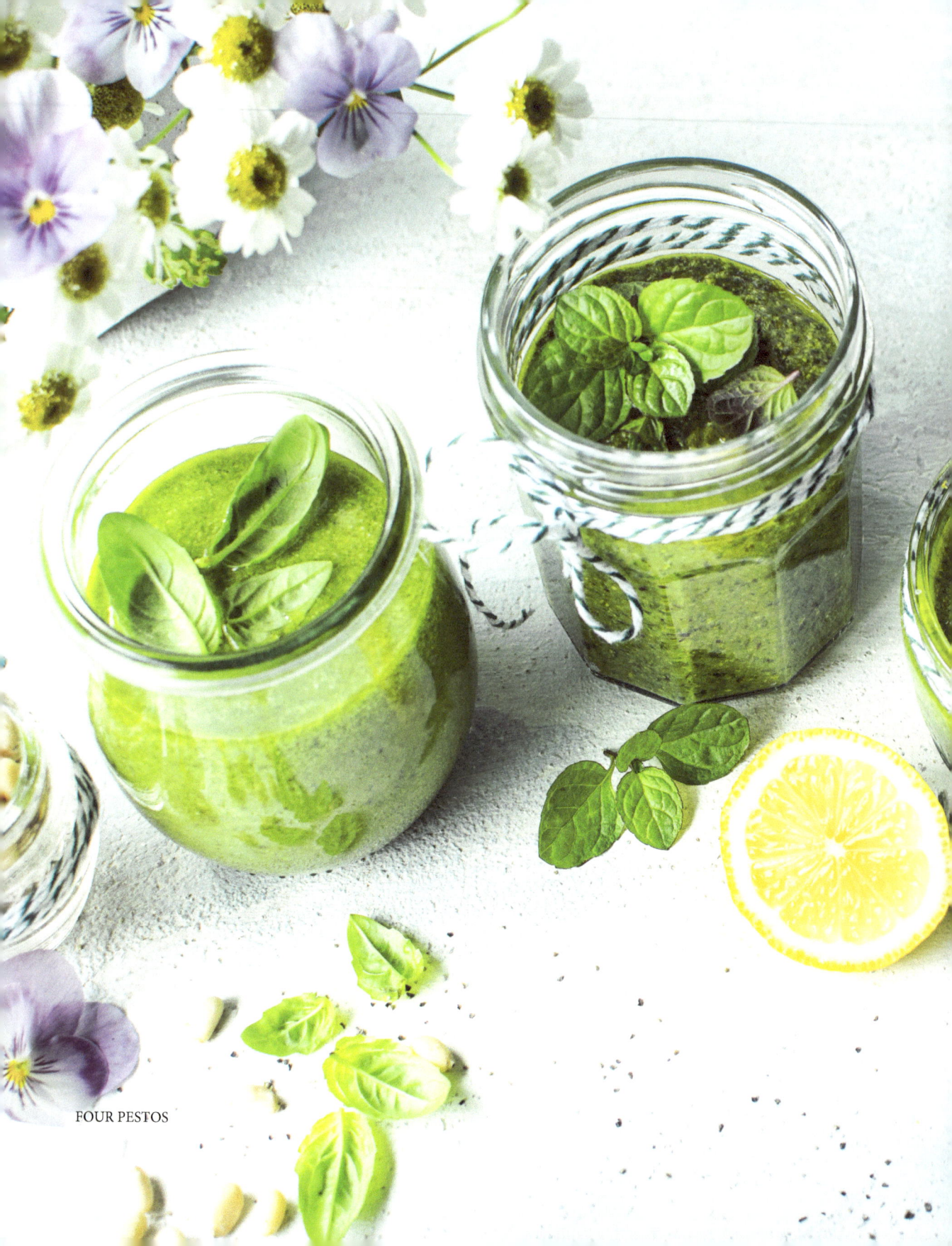

FOUR PESTOS

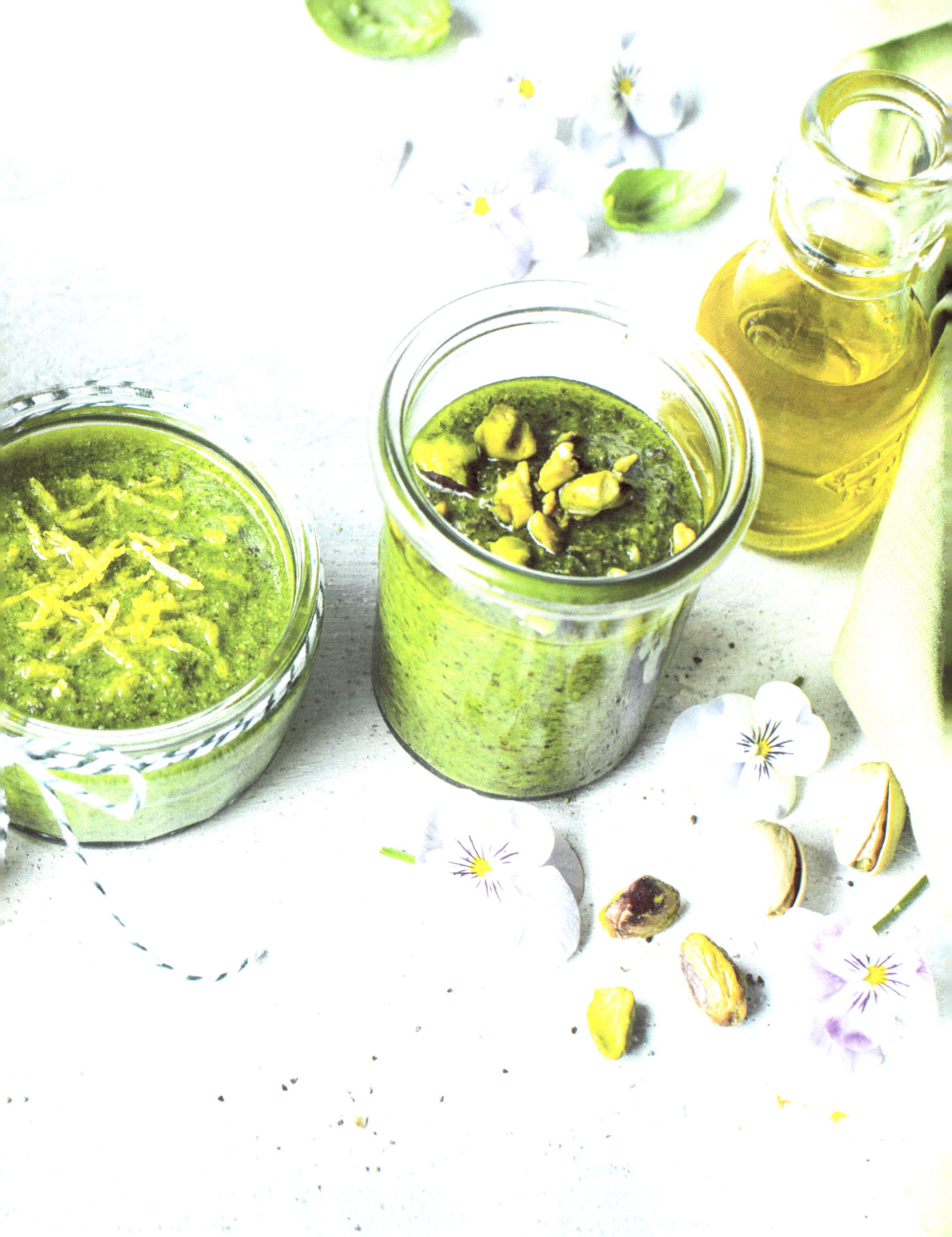

FOUR PESTOS

These pestos are great for pasta, salads, mixed with vegetables or used as toppings. Herbs are famous for their medicinal properties and there is no better way to consume them than fresh. Packed with vitamins, healthy fats and antioxidants and with them being such a quick and easy way to add flavour to a dish, these pesto's are always favourite go-to.

CLASSIC PESTO

20g fresh basil
40g pine nuts
3 tbsp nutritional yeast
1 raw garlic clove
8 tbsp olive oil
2 tbsp water
Salt

STEP 1
Place all ingredients into a blender and blend until desired consistency.

PISTACHIO PESTO

20g fresh basil
50g pistachio nuts w/o shell
8–10 tbsp olive oil
3 tbsp nutritional yeast
2 roasted garlic
2 tbsp water
Salt
Add a couple tbsp of coconut milk for creamy texture

STEP 1
Peel garlic and lightly drizzle with olive oil, roast in the oven for 10 minutes at 180 degrees.

STEP 2
Place all ingredients into a blender and blend until desired consistency.

MINT PESTO

40 fresh mint leaves
50g fresh almonds
8–10 tbsp olive oil
3 tbsp water
Half tsp Dijon mustard
Squeeze of lemon
2 roasted garlic
Salt

STEP 1
Peel garlic and lightly drizzle with olive oil, roast in the oven for 10 minutes at 180 degrees.

STEP 2
Place all ingredients into a blender and blend until desired consistency.

LEMON PESTO

20g fresh basil
1 raw garlic
3 tbsp nutritional yeast
40g pine nuts
½ lemon juice
¼ of the lemon's zest
7 tbsp olive oil
Salt
Pepper

STEP 1
Place all ingredients into a blender and blend until desired consistency.

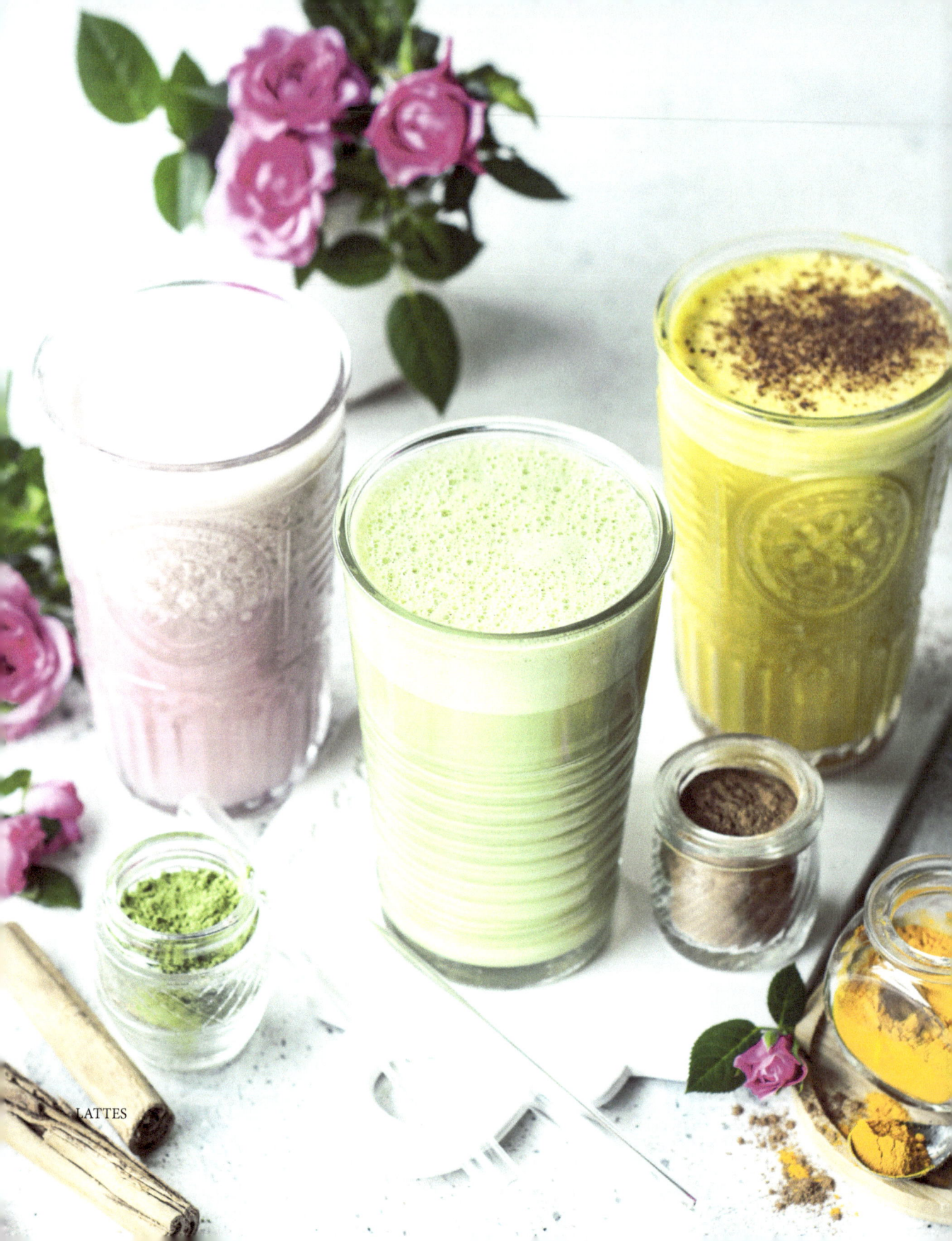

LATTES

LATTES

Choose a latte that suits your mood today. The rose latte is sweet and calming, rosewater is known to sooth the skin, treat infections and enhance mood. Matcha contains caffeine therefore giving us energy, but it also does things like boost brain function and speeds up the metabolism. Golden milk is famous for its medicinal purposes such as fighting inflammation, preventing cell damage, lowering blood sugar levels and boosting the immune system.

ROSE LATTE

SERVES 2 PEOPLE

500 ml almond milk
5 tbsp rosewater
3 cherries
1 tbsp maple syrup
1 vanilla bean
1 tbsp coconut oil

STEP 1
Pit the cherries then blend all the ingredients together.

STEP 2
In a saucepan heat the latte up, turning off before boiling.

MATCHA LATTE

SERVES 2 PEOPLE

2 tsp matcha powder
2 cup oat milk

1 tbsp hazelnut butter
2 tsp maple syrup
1 tsp cinnamon
2 tbsp coconut milk

STEP 1
Blend all the ingredients together.

STEP 2
In a saucepan heat the latte up, turning off before boiling.

GOLDEN MILK

SERVES 2 PEOPLE

1½ cup almond milk
1 cup light coconut milk from carton
1½ tsp ground turmeric
¼ tsp ground ginger
2 tbsp maple syrup
1 tbsp coconut oil
1 cinnamon stick

Pinch pepper
Small pinch salt
Ground cinnamon to sprinkle on top

STEP 1
Combine all the ingredients together in a saucepan and whisk until mixed.

STEP 2
Place the cinnamon stick in the saucepan and heat the latte up, turning off before boiling.

STEP 3
Remove the cinnamon stick, pour into cups and top with a sprinkle of ground cinnamon.

Acknowledgments

I would like to thank my family and friends for all the love and support they have shown me towards my new-found passion towards writing and cooking. I would like to thank my boyfriend for testing out all of my recipes with me first hand, and always being so supportive. Thank you to my food stylist and photographer Olympia Davis for working very closely with me on the image and display of the recipes in this book and doing such an amazing job with the pictures. And I would like to thank the universe for bringing me to this new venture, inspiring me through meditation and blessing me with the time and resources to learn and create.

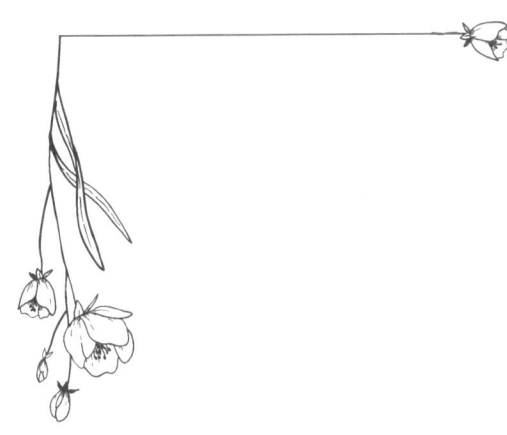

I treasure my body by eating natural foods and staying active

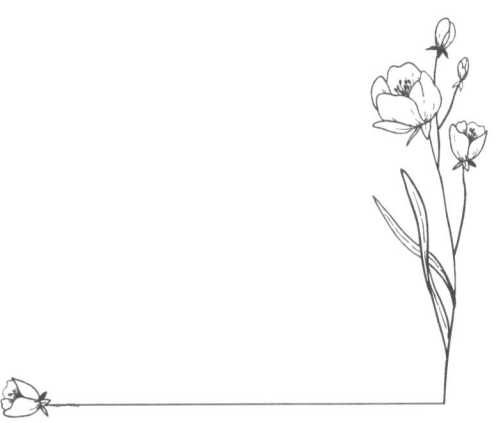

Lightning Source UK Ltd.
Milton Keynes UK
UKHW050750041022
409879UK00003B/54